Recovering from Depression

Recovering from Depression

A Workbook for Teens

Revised Edition

by

Mary Ellen Copeland, M.A., M.S.

and

Stuart Copans, M.D.

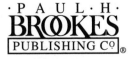

·P A U L·H·
BROOKES
PUBLISHING C⁰ ®

Baltimore • London • Sydney

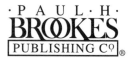

Paul H. Brookes Publishing Co.
Post Office Box 10624
Baltimore, Maryland 21285-0624

www.brookespublishing.com

Typeset by Integrated Publishing Solutions, Grand Rapids, Michigan.
Manufactured in the United States of America by
Versa Press, Inc., East Peoria, Illinois.

Third printing of revised edition, August 2007.

Cases described in this book are composites based on the authors' actual experiences.
Individuals' names have been changed and identifying details have been altered to
protect confidentiality.

Library of Congress Cataloging-in-Publication Data

Copeland, Mary Ellen.
   Recovering from depression : a workbook for teens / by Mary Ellen Copeland, Stuart
Copans.
      v. cm.
   Contents: Getting started — Things I need to know about my physical and
emotional health — Things I can do to help myself feel better — Things
I can do to maintain a positive outlook over the long term — Building
an ongoing recovery and safety plan.
   ISBN-13: 978-1-55766-592-8
   ISBN-10: 1-55766-592-3
     1. Depression in adolescence—Juvenile literature.   2. Teenagers—Mental health—
Juvenile literature. [1. Depression, Mental.]   I. Copans, Stuart.   II. Title.
RJ506.D4 C685 2002
616.85'27'00835—dc21
                                                      2002018291

British Library Cataloguing in Publication data are available from the British Library.

Contents

About the Authors

Mary Ellen Copeland, M.A., M.S., is a mental health educator. She has worked with adults and young people all over the world, teaching them how to recover from troubling conditions such as depression and how to stay well. She has also worked as a teacher, founding and directing a school for teens with special needs. Ms. Copeland believes that if teens understand how they feel and know how to help themselves feel well, they will be happier and better able to do the things they want to do.

Ms. Copeland received her master's degree in counseling psychology from Vermont College of Norwich University and her master's degree in resource management and administration from Antioch New England Graduate School.

Ms. Copeland is the author of

- *The Depression Workbook: A Guide for Living with Depression and Manic Depression*
- *Living Without Depression and Manic Depression: A Workbook for Maintaining Mood Stability*
- *Wellness Recovery Action Plan*
- *Winning Against Relapse: A Workbook of Action Plans for Recurring Health and Emotional Problems*
- *The Worry Control Workbook*
- *The Loneliness Workbook: A Guide to Developing and Maintaining Lasting Connections*
- *Healing the Trauma of Abuse: A Women's Workbook,* co-authored with Maxine Harris

Stuart Copans, M.D., is a husband, father, child psychiatrist, cartoonist, writer, speaker, book illustrator, paper cutter, bookplate designer, mail artist, book artist, swimmer, and canoe paddler (not always in that order). His children have all survived his parenting mistakes, for which he is grateful to them and to some undefined higher power. He enjoys collaborating with others and hopes they enjoy collaborating with him but always feels as if he's the lucky one in any collaboration.

Dr. Copans graduated magna cum laude from Harvard University and received his medical degree from Stanford Medical School. He has researched parent–child interactions for the National Institute of Child Health and Human Development and has worked with adolescents in both inpatient and outpatient settings for nearly 30 years. He is on the faculty of Dartmouth Medical School and the University of Massachusetts Medical School and is board certified in child and adolescent psychiatry.

Dr. Copans likes to write books that teach through humor or that help people deal with problems. His books include

- *Who's the Patient Here?: Portraits of the Young Psychotherapist,* co-authored with Thomas Singer

- *How to Avoid the Evil Eye,* by Brenda Rosenbaum

- *Smart Moves: Your Guide Through the Emotional Maze of Relocation,* co-authored with Audrey McCollum and Nadia Jensen

- *Twelve Jewish Steps to Recovery: A Personal Guide to Turning from Alcoholism and Other Addictions,* co-authored with Rabbi Kerry Olitzky

- *The Healing Journey: Your Journal of Self-Discovery,* co-authored with Phil Rich

- *The Healing Journey for Couples: Your Journal of Mutual Discovery,* co-authored with Phil Rich

- *The Healing Journey Through Addiction: Your Journal for Recovery and Self-Renewal,* co-authored with Phil Rich

- *The Healing Journey Through Job Loss: Your Journal for Reflection and Revitalization,* co-authored with Phil Rich and Kenneth G. Copans

Acknowledgments

Thank you to my husband, Ed, for his editorial and personal support as this book moved to fruition. I also thank my children and all of the young people whose lives have touched mine and who have made me want to write this book.

Mary Ellen Copeland

Thank you to all of the adolescent patients who field-tested this book for us and also the adolescents and parents who helped me learn about adolescent depression through their honesty and sharing. I also thank Nick Belsky, who continues to inspire me through his ability to help families help their adolescents, and Phil Rich, who helped expand my knowledge of how journaling can help adolescents and their families. This book has benefited from our work with the team that helped develop a high school wellness curriculum to accompany this book. Finally, I thank my co-author, Mary Ellen, for her patience and perseverance and for her willingness to adapt her pioneering work on self-management of depression in adults to help adolescents and to try to reach those adolescents who don't yet realize that help is available and that they can feel better.

Stuart Copans

To young people all over the world
in the hope that this book will give them
the tools and strategies they need to be
healthy, happy, and successful
in whatever they want to do

Introduction

This book was written to help you if you are a young person who is having a hard time with things like

- Experiencing long periods of sadness
- Thinking about hurting yourself
- Feeling isolated from your friends
- Not enjoying or dropping out of activities that used to make you feel good about yourself
- Being irritable and angry most of the time
- Feeling you have no control over bad things that are happening to you

It is written with the understanding that

1. Depression goes away. If you help yourself as much as possible, you will feel better faster, and it is more likely that you will stay well. You can also benefit from reaching out for assistance and support from family members, friends, and health care providers.

2. There are many causes of depression, but usually depression is brought on by a combination of several factors, including chemical changes in the body and life experiences. Regardless of where depression comes from, there are many things that you and others can do to help you feel better.

3. Depression can tell you that you need to change something in your way of living, but when depression gets too deep, it is no longer a help, but a danger, and you will need to help yourself and get help from others.

how this book is organized

This book is organized into five sections:

1. Getting Started
2. Things I Need to Know About My Physical and Emotional Health
3. Things I Can Do to Help Myself Feel Better
4. Things I Can Do to Maintain a Positive Outlook over the Long Term
5. Building an Ongoing Recovery and Safety Plan

Each section contains a number of chapters, with each chapter focusing on one specific area. There are also four appendixes in the back that include helpful telephone numbers and information for parents and friends.

We have shared this book with a number of young people like you, and they have found it to be helpful. We hope it is helpful to you. Please let us know what you think and suggest ways we could improve this book so that it is even more helpful to teenagers with depression. Check out our web site at **http://www. brookespublishing.com/recovering** where you will find an updated list of important telephone numbers (as found in Appendix C) and a copy of the questionnaire found in the back of the book. You can mail in the questionnaire or fill out an on-line version. You can also check out Mary Ellen Copeland's web site at **http://www.mentalhealthrecovery.com** to find articles, information, and resources on mental health and depression. Keep checking the web sites for exciting new features!

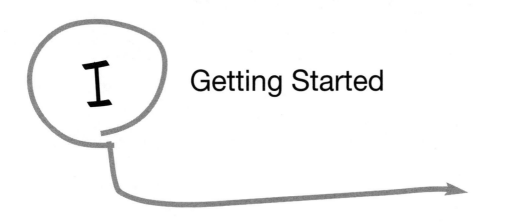

Getting Started

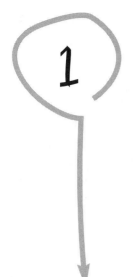

Am I Depressed?

overview

Have you been feeling really awful and don't know why? If so, you may be depressed. Many people are depressed, don't know they are depressed, and don't know why they feel so bad. You deserve to feel well. Your health and happiness are important. If you are depressed, you can help yourself to feel better, and you can get help from others. This book will give you information to help you do that.

information

The Depression Survey on pages 4–6 will help you discover if you are depressed. But before you take this survey, answer the following questions. Have you been:

_____ Feeling like killing yourself?

_____ Making plans as to how you will kill yourself?

_____ Wishing you were dead?

_____ Wishing you would get killed accidentally?

_____ Feeling like killing yourself is the only way to solve your problems?

DO NOT ACT ON THESE FEELINGS. GET HELP RIGHT NOW.

If you answered yes to any of these questions, you need help right away. Turn immediately to Chapter 3, *Suicide Prevention.*

things to remember

1. If you are feeling bad, even if you are not sure whether or not it is depression, don't use alcohol or street drugs to make yourself feel better. They will make you feel better at first, but you will feel much worse later. Street drugs and alcohol can keep you from seeking the help you need to really feel better, and they often lead to an addiction, which can be a very big problem.

2. You may think you will never feel better, but you will. Depression ends. By helping yourself and getting help from others, you will begin feeling much better very soon.

3. It is not your fault you feel this way. Don't blame yourself. That will just make you feel worse.

> *Every morning my mother tries to get me up to go to school. I feel so awful. I don't want to get up. I just want to keep my head under the covers and sleep all day. If I go to school, I know I will fail. I'm sure I will flunk that math test. I can't understand anything the teachers are saying anyway. None of my friends like me anymore. I used to like the Drama Club, but now I can't stand it. Everyone is laughing and having a good time, and I'm not part of it. I don't think anyone even cares about me.*

The following checklist will help you discover for yourself if you are depressed. Check off any symptoms that apply to you.

depression survey

DO YOU FEEL:

_____ Hopeless, worthless, useless, like not caring about anything, like you might as well be dead, like you are a failure?

_____ That there is no solution to your problems?

_____ Numb, without feelings?

_____ Like you have nothing to look forward to?

_____ Like you never have any fun?

_____ Ugly, like everyone is staring at you?

_____ Like nobody would miss you if you were gone?

_____ Like sleeping all the time or sleeping much more than 8 hours a day; or you have trouble sleeping and seem to be awake all night?

_____ Like you don't want to eat anything or like eating all the time?

_____ Very tired almost all the time?

_____ Irritable, angry, and/or anxious most of the time?

_____ Like you don't want to do anything?

_____ Very lonely, even when you are with your friends or family?

_____ Like you are a bad person?

_____ Like there is no one you can trust or talk to, that no one likes or cares about you?

HAVE YOU:

_____ Lost more than 10 pounds recently without being on a diet (you just don't feel like eating)?

_____ Secretly cut, burned, or hurt yourself?

_____ Heard your friends telling you they are worried about you, that you are quieter than usual, or that you are always in a bad mood?

DO YOU:

_____ Have a hard time getting up in the morning or find you are unable to get up for school or work?

_____ Worry a lot?

_____ Have a very negative attitude?

_____ Cry easily?

ARE YOU:

_____ Very quiet?

_____ Always thinking about mistakes you have made in the past?

DO YOU TRY TO HIDE THE WAY YOU FEEL BY:

_____ Smiling when you don't feel like it?

_____ Taking risks such as driving too fast?

_____ Having sex?

———— Using drugs and alcohol?

———— Getting in fights?

———— Secretly hurting yourself?

———— Not showing your feelings?

things to do

You need to get help for depression right away if you:

- Checked off or answered yes to several of the symptoms of depression
- Have felt bad for more than 2 weeks
- Feel so bad you can't keep up with your schoolwork and other responsibilities
- Are thinking about hurting or killing yourself or anyone else
- Think a lot about dying

things to remember

The next chapter will tell you how to get help. Don't delay. Get help now. You deserve to feel better. The sooner you get help, the sooner you will feel better.

After you have gotten help, there are things you can do to help yourself feel better and to keep you from getting depressed again. But first, get help.

Do not turn to alcohol or street drugs to make you feel better. They will make you feel better for a very short time, but after the effects wear off, you will feel MUCH WORSE.

next steps

If you think a friend is depressed, turn to Appendix A, *If a Friend Is Depressed,* to find out what to do.

2 Getting Help

overview

If the first chapter revealed that you are depressed, *you need help, support, and good advice right away.* When you're depressed, it is often very hard to reach out and get help. But it is worth the effort. This chapter will help guide you through the process of getting help.

information

You need at least one person, but it is best if you have several people who:

- Understand how you are feeling
- Can stay with you
- Will listen to you
- Will help you find help from health care providers

> My friend Miranda keeps asking me what's wrong and why I don't want to hang out anymore. She says she thinks I'm sick. She even told me she was going to tell my parents that something is wrong with me, but I begged her not to. They don't even notice how bad I feel. They would probably just get mad at me.

You may feel as if you have no one you can really tell, but you are not alone. Many people of all ages feel that way. Feeling scared to talk to people is part of depression. If you have no one you can talk to, read this chapter on how to get help for yourself. When you have gotten help and are feeling better, read Chapter 9, *Friends and Supporters.*

things to do

Who can you tell? You probably feel most comfortable talking to your friends. Telling an understanding friend that you are depressed is fine. However, because depression is a very serious problem and other people your age may not know anything about it, it is best to *rely on a trusted adult to get you the help you need.*

Seek out people who can give you good advice, help, and support. If you tell a peer that you are depressed and they give you some advice, use your own judgment to decide if it is good advice. Don't give in to pressure from others who are giving you bad advice or advice that doesn't feel right to you. Examples of *bad advice*:

- "Try drinking or street drugs. They'll make you feel better."
- "Pack up your things and run away from home."
- "Drive your car really fast to give yourself a thrill."
- "Get a boyfriend (girlfriend)."

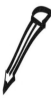

questions to answer

Other examples of bad advice I have gotten from friends:

_____

_____

_____

_____

information

Who are the adults in your life who may be able to help you and give you good advice about dealing with your depression?

They are people who will:

- Listen to you
- Let you know they are supportive of you
- Help you figure out what to do
- Get help for you if you ask them to
- Keep what you tell them private unless they need to share the information to keep you safe
- Get help for you if they think you are in danger, even if you don't ask them

It is NOT HELPFUL if they:

- Blame you (tell you it is your fault)
- Give you bad or wrong advice like "Just pull yourself together, and get over it."
- Criticize you
- Judge you
- Tease or taunt you
- Treat you badly
- Threaten you
- Punish you

Don't give up too easily on people who could help you. Some people will change the way they treat you if you *tell them what you need and what you don't need.*

The person you ask to help could be:

- Parent or parents*
- Your family doctor*
- Counselor, therapist, or health care provider*
- School counselor*
- School nurse or school doctor*
- Minister, priest, rabbi, youth minister, or other religious counselor*
- Older brother or sister
- Aunt, uncle, cousin, or grandparent
- Teacher
- Family friend

(*Best choices if you trust them and they treat you well)

FINDING SOMEONE TO TELL CAN BE VERY HARD. DON'T GIVE UP. YOU ARE WORTH IT!

things to do

People I am going to tell how I feel and ask for help:

_____

_____

_____

_____

_____

_____

information

You may decide that one person is the best person to tell and that he or she will be able to give you the kind of support, advice, and assistance you need. Then, when you actually tell the person, you find that she or he is critical of you, or you feel that he or she treats you harshly or is inappropriate in some way. *They were wrong, not you. Don't blame yourself. Tell someone else.*

working with your parents

When you are depressed, you may find that it becomes hard to ask for help from other people, especially your parents. However, your parents may be the best people to help you get the help you need. In addition, you may need their support for payment and insurance as you obtain medical assistance.

things to do

Show your parents Appendix B, *Information for Parents*. It will help them to understand what you are going through. You may want to share with them other information in this book. To prepare for talking with your parents you will need to decide:

- If you want to tell them individually or when they are together
- What you want to tell them

information

You have had a close relationship with your parents for a long time. We hope it's been a good relationship, that you can tell them exactly how you are feeling, and that you would like them to help you get help for dealing with your depression. If it is a good relationship, they will respond with loving support and suggestions. If you are thinking about hurting yourself, it is important that you let them know. If you have tried to hurt yourself in the past, it is important to let them know that, too.

If your relationship with your parents is not good, you will need to think about how much you can tell them and how much help you can expect them to give you. Then, you will have to reach out to other trusted adults, like those listed in this chapter, to assist you in getting the help you need.

things to do

If you can't think of any adult you trust enough to tell, you are not alone. Many people feel that they don't have anyone in their lives they can trust, especially when they are depressed. Also, many adults, even family members, are too busy to establish good supportive relationships with the younger people in their lives. This is too bad. You may end up feeling isolated and lonely. That doesn't mean something is wrong with you. It means something is wrong with our society. You deserve to have caring, supportive adults in your life.

There are adults who care. You may not have come into contact with them yet. You may have to do some detective work to find them. This may be hard for you when you are depressed. Try to do it anyway! Where to look for help:

1. Try your telephone book. Most telephone books have a guide to services in the pages at the front. There are several places you can look for help on that page, or look under *Health* and *Mental Health* in the Yellow Pages. You will find numbers for:

- The local informational *hotline,* with volunteers who answer the telephone and can tell you how to get help

- Emergency counseling or mental health numbers that will be able to direct you to help

- Hospitals that provide special services for people who are depressed

- Your local general hospital (they should be able to direct you to help)

2. There are several national organizations that can direct you to help in your area. Those telephone numbers are listed in Appendix C, *Important Telephone Numbers.*

3. If this research is too much for you, call the operator and ask for the number of the emergency hotline.

If one source doesn't work out, try another. Calls made to these services are always strictly confidential. You don't have to worry that the person who answers will tell anyone else unless you ask them to. However, if they feel you might hurt yourself or someone else, they may be required by law to tell someone who can help you and protect you.

If you are having trouble reaching one of these agencies, refer to Chapter 4, *Helping Myself Feel Better Right Away,* for things you can do to help yourself while you are trying to get other assistance. Remember, you will feel good again.

things to remember

When you have found someone to help you, what do you tell them? Tell the person you choose that:

1. You are depressed.

2. You have been depressed for _____ (how long).

3. You have learned that this is very serious, and you need help right away.

4. They need to assist you in finding help because you are too depressed to do it yourself.

5. They have to stay with you or arrange for someone else to stay with you if you are feeling like killing yourself. (See Chapter 3, *Suicide Prevention.*)

6. They will have to do things for you that you would usually do for yourself if you were feeling well, like making telephone calls and arranging transportation to appointments, keeping in touch with your teachers, and getting your homework assignments. *Ask clearly for what you need, even though it is hard.*

things to do

INSIST THAT YOU GET HELP RIGHT AWAY. DON'T WAIT!

If you wait, the depression may worsen. If you are told to wait several days, tell the care provider you need help NOW. Don't get off the line or stop talking with someone until you have gotten an appointment right away or have been referred to other sources of help. If you can't get to the appointment yourself, ask them to arrange transportation for you.

next steps

After you have gotten help for yourself, turn to Chapter 4, *Helping Myself Feel Better Right Away,* and to Chapter 5, *Using the Rest of this Book,* to increase your understanding of depression, to learn how to get the support you need, and to find out how to keep from getting depressed again.

3 Suicide Prevention

questions to answer

Have you been:

____ Feeling like killing yourself?

____ Making plans as to how you will kill yourself?

____ Wishing you were dead?

____ Wishing you would get killed accidentally?

____ Feeling like killing yourself is the only way to solve your problems?

If you answered yes to any of these questions, continue to work your way through this chapter. If you answered no to all of these questions, you can skip over this chapter.

things to do

DO NOT HURT YOURSELF! GET HELP RIGHT NOW.

TALK TO PEOPLE! CALL PEOPLE! SCREAM! YELL!

DO WHATEVER YOU HAVE TO DO
TO MAKE SOMEONE WHO CAN HELP HEAR YOU!

YOU ARE WORTH IT! YOU CAN START TO FEEL BETTER SOON!

> *I was really going to do it this time. I had been thinking about it for a long time. Things are never going to get any better. But I started thinking about my dog. I am the only one in my family who cares about Pete. Nobody else will take him for a walk into the mountains. He loves to smell everything. Nobody else will toss a stick for him or play Frisbee with him.*

If you kill yourself, you can never:

- Raise a family
- Go for a ride on a motorcycle
- Swim in the ocean
- Go to a concert by your favorite musicians
- Eat another bowl of your favorite ice cream
- Watch the sun set
- Ride on a roller coaster

If you kill yourself, you'll never do any of the things you dream about doing.

Some of the big and little things I look forward to doing:

_____

_____

_____

_____

_____

_____

keep yourself safe

Tell a trusted adult exactly how you are feeling. Do this right away. Don't read any further until you have done this. The person you ask to help could be:

- Parent or parents*
- Your family doctor*

- Counselor, therapist, or mental health professional*
- School counselor*
- School nurse or school physician*
- Minister, priest, rabbi or other religious counselor*
- Older brother or sister
- Aunt, uncle, cousin, or grandparent
- Teacher
- Family friend

(*Best choices if they meet the criteria listed in Chapter 2, *Getting Help*)

If none of these people is appropriate or you can't reach the person, call:

- Local police
- Hospital emergency room
- Community mental health center emergency service
- Local hotline or teen hotline
- 911, if you have this service in your area
- One of the telephone numbers listed in Appendix C, *Important Telephone Numbers*

Telephone books have emergency numbers for the local police and hospital emergency room inside the front cover, and the telephone numbers of crisis services like the local mental health emergency center or local hotline on the information page. If you can't find an adult to tell, refer to Chapter 2, *Getting Help*, to get more information and advice on how to find someone to tell. Make sure the person you tell believes you. That person should make sure you are never alone and should help you find ongoing support and assistance. If the person you tell doesn't believe you or says you are just trying to get attention, yell, scream—do whatever you have to do to get them to listen to you and take action.

- Do not be alone under any circumstance.
- Do not use alcohol or street drugs. They increase the risk of suicide. (If you are a habitual user of either drugs or alcohol, see Chapter 10, *Avoiding Substance Abuse*, for information on how to get help.)
- Do not proceed beyond this point until you have gotten help for yourself and are no longer feeling suicidal.

next steps

After you have dealt with this very dangerous situation, there are some things you can do to keep this from ever happening again.

1. Some teenagers commit suicide because a bad thing has happened, like they got a poor grade, they are pregnant, they broke the law, their boyfriend or girlfriend broke up with them, someone made fun of them or humiliated them, or they are having a hard time getting along with their parents. These situations are very painful. *But suicide is never a good solution to these problems.* Suicide is a permanent solution to a temporary problem. It doesn't solve anything. Family members and friends will be haunted by this event for the rest of their lives. And you won't do all the wonderful things you have dreamed of doing. For help in finding solutions to problems, turn to Chapter 11, *When Bad Things Happen.*

2. Train your brain not to think of suicide as a solution to your problems. Do not allow yourself to think suicidal thoughts. See Chapter 17, *Changing Negative Thoughts to Positive Ones.* Some examples of suicidal thoughts and their positive responses are:

Negative thought	Positive response
"I want to die."	"I choose to live."
"Suicide is the only way out of this bad situation."	"There are many solutions to this problem. Some of them may be hard, but I can work my way through them."
"Everybody will be better off with me dead."	"Everyone wants me to live."
"I can't deal with these painful feelings."	"Painful feelings fade over time and eventually go away."

3. Be aware of the things that make you feel like ending your life. Then, you can try to avoid those situations or plan something fun to do or people to be with during hard times. For example, you may notice that you feel more suicidal in the evening because that is the time of day you spent with your girlfriend before she broke up with you. You could arrange to play basketball with a group of your friends every day at that time. Or use that time to play a musical instru-

ment, talk to a good friend, read a book, write in your journal, or paint a picture. If being with certain people makes you feel bad about yourself, avoid those people and spend time with people who make you feel good about yourself.

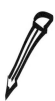

questions to answer

I FEEL WORSE:

- *Time of day*

    _____ When I first get up

    _____ In the morning

    _____ In the afternoon

    _____ At dinnertime

    _____ In the evening

- *During the holiday season.* Many people feel more suicidal around the holiday season. Maybe it is because everyone else seems to be having such a good time and you feel awful.

    I feel worse around the holidays. Which holidays?

    _____

    _____

    _____

    _____

    _____

- *During certain seasons.* If you notice you are more depressed and have suicidal thoughts in the fall and winter, refer to the "Light" section of Chapter 12, *Diet, Light, Exercise, and Sleep.* If you notice you are more depressed and suicidal in the summer, do what you can to keep cool, such as staying in air-conditioned rooms, going swimming, or taking a cool bath or shower.

    I notice I feel more depressed:

    _____ In the fall and winter

    _____ In the spring and summer

- *On or around anniversary dates of traumatic experiences or the loss of a loved one.* Be aware that it is common for everyone to feel more depressed and even suicidal on these anniversary dates.

  Anniversary dates that make me feel more depressed:

  Date and event

  _____   _____

  Date and event

  _____   _____

  Date and event

  _____   _____

  Date and event

  _____   _____

  Plan ahead for these hard days. Spend them with people you enjoy and/or doing things you love to do. Treat yourself like the special person you are to help you get through this hard time.

- *At certain places.* They can also bring up memories of events that were traumatizing or the loss of a loved one.

  Places that trigger suicidal thoughts:

  _____

  _____

  _____

  _____

  _____

  _____

  _____

  _____

  Avoid these places as much as possible. Take along a supportive friend for those times when you must be there.

- *Around certain people.*

  People who make me feel suicidal:

  _____

  _____

  _____

  _____

  _____

  _____

Know who they are, and avoid them as much as possible. Spend as much time as you can with people who help you to feel good about yourself.

things to do

When these triggers come up, be prepared. Take the following action:

- Spend time with good friends and supportive people.
- Engage in an activity you enjoy, like shooting hoops, playing music, or watching a fun video.
- Do everything you can to take good care of yourself—exercise, get plenty of outdoor light, eat healthy food, and limit your intake of sugar and caffeine.

next steps

Refer to Chapter 4, *Helping Myself Feel Better Right Away*, for more ideas on how to help yourself through hard times.

Deal with depression when you first notice early warning signs rather than when the symptoms have gotten very severe. Refer to Chapter 19, *Monitoring My Moods and Preventing Depression.*

Keep Yourself Safe by Developing a Safety Plan

Once you have gotten rid of suicidal feelings, you might think you will never feel that way again. However, to be sure to keep yourself safe, it is good to do some advance planning and preparation just in case those feelings ever do come up again.

things to do

Make a commitment to yourself and other people in your life that you will never try to take your own life. Fill in the following form. Copy it, and give it to all your supporters. Ideas for things you might want others to do are listed below.

I, _____ (your name),
promise myself and those of you I love that I will never try to
end my life. If I am having suicidal thoughts, I will tell one of
you. If I tell you or if you think I am in danger of ending my life,
I want you to:

_____

_____

_____

_____

_____

_____

I want you to take this action even if I tell you not to, even if I
get mad at you. It may be necessary to save my life.

Signed: _____

Date: _____

Ideas of action you could ask others to take include:

- Calling your parents, a trusted adult, 911, emergency services, your doctor, or your counselor
- Staying with you or arranging to have someone with you at all times

- Listening to you and letting you talk or cry or be angry for as long as necessary
- Physically preventing you from doing anything to harm yourself
- Taking you to the hospital
- Diverting your attention with good videos
- Keeping you from watching violent or disturbing television shows, videos, or movies

Have emergency telephone numbers and telephone numbers of close friends and family members posted in a convenient place so that when you are feeling suicidal you can easily call someone. It is very difficult to find telephone numbers or even to remember who to call when you are feeling suicidal.

Copy the following card, fill in the telephone numbers, and keep it near your telephone.

---

emergency telephone number list

Doctor	_____
Counselor	_____
Police	_____
Hotline	_____
Emergency services	_____
911	

Make a small card to carry in your pocket that lists important telephone numbers and things you can do to keep yourself safe. Cut out the following card, glue it to a heavier piece of paper, and carry it in your wallet, pocket, or purse; or make your own card, revising it in any way that would make it more useful to you. Add a trusted friend, grandparent, or other relative under "Other."

Telephone numbers of people to call if I am feeling desperate
or suicidal:

Mother at work ＿＿＿＿＿＿   Father at work ＿＿＿＿＿＿

At home ＿＿＿＿＿＿＿＿   At home ＿＿＿＿＿＿＿＿

Emergency
services ＿＿＿＿＿＿＿＿   Police ＿＿＿＿＿＿＿＿＿

Doctor ＿＿＿＿＿＿＿＿   Counselor ＿＿＿＿＿＿＿

Other:
Name ＿＿＿＿＿＿＿＿＿   Number ＿＿＿＿＿＿＿＿

Hotlines ＿＿＿＿＿＿＿＿＿＿＿＿＿＿＿＿＿＿＿＿

911

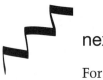

next steps

For more information on developing a safety plan, refer to Chapter 20,
Developing a Safety Plan. If you think a friend might be suicidal or know
your friend is suicidal, turn to Appendix A, *If a Friend Is Depressed.*

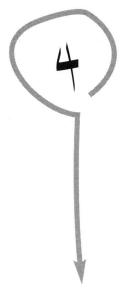

Helping Myself
Feel Better Right Away

overview

Although the most important thing you can do when you realize you are depressed is to get help, there are some simple things you can do to help yourself feel a little better—and some things you should avoid doing. However, *they do not take the place of getting help right away.*

> *I keep thinking about how bad I feel and wishing there was something I could do to help myself feel better. I tried drinking. I felt really good after I had a couple of beers a few weeks ago. I forgot about my problems and even laughed a few times. But since I'm not 21, it's such a hassle to get it. And if I get caught with it, I will be in more trouble than I am now. There must be something else I can do. I think I'll go shoot a few hoops and see if that makes me feel any better.*

Following are some things that won't help—things that will definitely make you feel worse in the short and long run.

things to avoid

- Drinking alcohol. Even though it makes you feel better at first, you will feel worse later.
- Taking street drugs or any medications that are not prescribed by *your own* doctor
- Having sex indiscriminately

- Doing anything careless or reckless

- Making any major decisions until you feel better—like leaving home or dropping out of school while you are depressed

- Watching the news or other shows on television with a lot of violence

- Spending time with people who are judgmental, critical, make you feel bad about yourself, try to pick fights, harass you, ridicule you, blame you, or try to shame you

- Eating junk food that is loaded with sugar, fat, salt, and additives (candy, cookies, cake, donuts, chips, fries, soda, and so forth). For more information on diet see Chapter 12, *Diet, Light, Exercise, and Sleep.*

information

The following ideas are *especially important if you are having a hard time getting help.* They may be difficult to do. When you are depressed, everything takes extra effort, but if you can do one or two of these things, it will help you feel a little better.

things to do

- Get together with one or several people who you really like. Avoid being alone until you feel better. This one is most important. *Do it even if you don't feel like it.* If you can't find anyone to be with, you could watch television or a video, listen to music, play with a pet, or read a story to a younger sibling.

- Get up at the same time each morning. People with depression agree that it makes them feel worse to stay in bed longer than usual. If you are really tired, take a short nap in the afternoon.

- Do an activity that involves movement, such as playing tennis; running; swimming; biking; aerobics; hiking; dancing; canoeing; working out on weight machines; playing soccer, volleyball, football, or baseball.

- Eat something healthy that you like, such as a bowl of cereal (not sugar coated), a sandwich, a salad, Chinese food, or pizza.

- Spend time doing something you enjoy, like watching sitcoms or a funny video, going to a movie, reading a comic, reading a light novel, playing video games, listening to music, making music (playing the guitar, piano, drums—whatever you enjoy), painting, drawing, working with clay, sculpting, building something, making jewelry, sewing, knitting, writing, cooking, or playing with a pet.

- Do something nice for someone else: help your parents with chores around the house, call or send a note to an elderly relative, or stop and visit someone at a nursing home or hospital.

Use the following space to write down some other things that you think might help you feel better.

Other things I enjoy doing that might help me feel better:

_____

_____

_____

_____

_____

The ideas in this chapter are useful:

- To temporarily divert you from how you feel
- After you are feeling better, to *keep* yourself feeling better
- Whenever you feel like you might be starting to feel depressed again

next steps

Refer to Chapter 5, *Using the Rest of this Book*, to decide what to do next on your journey to get rid of depression and to keep it away.

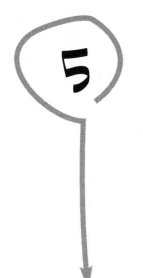

Using the Rest of this Book

overview

Now that you have gotten some of the help you need by working through Section I, *Getting Started:*

- Chapter 1: Am I Depressed?
- Chapter 2: Getting Help
- Chapter 3: Suicide Prevention
- Chapter 4: Helping Myself Feel Better Right Away

You can make some choices about how you want to use the rest of the book. You may want to read some of the information right away. You may prefer to read some of it later. You may have no interest in some of it.

things to remember

- You don't have to read the chapters in order.
- Read what seems most important to you right now.

If you can only read or work on a little bit at a time, that is fine. Do whatever you can. When you are depressed, it will be more difficult to work through this book. You will notice that as you start to feel better it will get easier.

next steps

Take a few minutes to read over this list of chapter contents. Number the chapters in the order you wish to read them. Then cross them off when you have finished them.

SECTION II: THINGS I NEED TO KNOW
ABOUT MY PHYSICAL AND EMOTIONAL HEALTH

_____ Chapter 6: Understanding Depression

_____ Chapter 7: Getting Good Health Care

_____ Chapter 8: Medication

SECTION III: THINGS I CAN DO TO HELP MYSELF FEEL BETTER

_____ Chapter 9: Friends and Supporters

_____ Chapter 10: Avoiding Substance Abuse

_____ Chapter 11: When Bad Things Happen

_____ Chapter 12: Diet, Light, Exercise, and Sleep

_____ Chapter 13: Helping Myself Relax

_____ Chapter 14: Peer Counseling

_____ Chapter 15: Creative Activities

SECTION IV: THINGS I CAN DO TO MAINTAIN
A POSITIVE OUTLOOK OVER THE LONG TERM

_____ Chapter 16: Raising Self-Esteem

_____ Chapter 17: Changing Negative Thoughts to Positive Ones

SECTION V: BUILDING AN ONGOING RECOVERY AND SAFETY PLAN

_____ Chapter 18: Wellness Tools

_____ Chapter 19: Monitoring My Moods and Preventing Depression

_____ Chapter 20: Developing a Safety Plan

_____ Chapter 21: Managing Medications

_____ Chapter 22: Avoiding Relapse

_____ Chapter 23: Dreams and Goals

APPENDIXES:

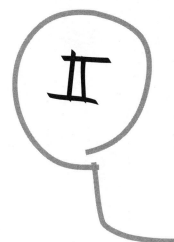

Things I Need to Know About My Physical and Emotional Health

6 Understanding Depression

I feel so awful. I feel like I am the worst person in the world. I don't know why I was ever born. It must be my fault. I must be doing something wrong. Why do I feel so miserable?

information

You may be interested in knowing some basic scientific facts and theories about depression. The part of the brain responsible for regulating emotions is call the *limbic system*. This area lies deep within the brain, below the *cerebrum*, which is the thinking part of the brain. In addition to emotions, the limbic system controls such functions as body temperature, appetite, hormone levels, sleep, blood pressure, and behavior.

Information is transmitted from one part of the brain to another with the help of a particular group of chemicals called *neurotransmitters*. This communication network is very delicately balanced. For the limbic system to perform properly, it is essential that this balance be maintained.

Two mechanisms within the limbic system allow signals to be passed from cell to cell. The first mechanism is *electrical stimulation*. An electrical impulse is generated in one nerve cell, or *neuron*, and travels down the length of the cell until it reaches a very small space or gap between that cell and the next (neurons are not really connected to each other). This gap between neurons is called a *synapse*. For information to be transmitted, the electrical impulse from the first cell must somehow get across the synapse to the next cell. But it can't jump across this space. Another mechanism is needed to transfer the electrical charge to the next cell.

Here, a second chemical mechanism comes into play. As the electrical impulse reaches the end of the first cell, it initiates a chemical reaction. A small sack containing neurotransmitters fuses with the cell wall. The sack then opens and empties the chemicals it contains into the gap between the cells. These chemicals float over to the second cell, attaching to the cell wall at specific places called *receptor sites.* Each receptor site will only accept a chemical that is the right shape to fit that site. When enough of the receptor sites are filled on the second cell, an *electrical impulse* is generated, which travels down this cell until it reaches the next synapse. There, the process is repeated. Electrical impulses travel from cell to cell in this manner throughout the limbic system and the rest of the central nervous system as well. The *hypothalamus,* located within the limbic system, serves as a sort of traffic controller.

Exactly what information is transmitted depends on which neurons are electrically activated and which part of the brain is stimulated by these neurons. When neural cells lose the ability to make the proper amount of a neurotransmitter, to store it properly, or bind it efficiently, depression may result.

A variety of factors are thought to affect neurotransmitter production and activity, including:

- Specific illnesses (that is why you need a complete physical examination if you are depressed)

- Hormonal imbalances

- Genetics (you inherited the tendency toward this problem)

- Stress (any kind of serious problem you have had or are having in your life. Refer to Chapter 11, *When Bad Things Happen,* and to Chapter 13, *Helping Myself Relax.*)

- Prescription and over-the-counter medications

- Illegal drug or alcohol use

- Seasonal Affective Disorder (See Chapter 12, *Diet, Light, Exercise, and Sleep.*)

- Poor diet (See Chapter 12, *Diet, Light, Exercise, and Sleep.*)

One or several of these factors may be causing or contributing to your depression. Although it is not possible to know precisely the contribution of each factor, it is useful to make a guess and to get others who know you to make guesses, too, because having some sense of the cause can help you figure out what to do to feel better.

Based on their assessment of the causes of your depression, your health care professionals will help you come up with a plan to reduce your symptoms and help you feel better as quickly as possible.

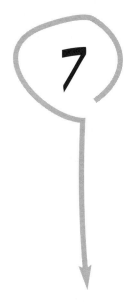

Getting Good Health Care

overview

In searching for relief from your symptoms of depression, you and your parents or other adults that are helping you can reach out to health care providers for assistance in helping you feel better.

> *My parents are really upset. The school nurse called and told them she was concerned about me, that she thought I might be depressed. I wish she would mind her own business. My parents started asking me all these questions. I don't feel like telling them anything. They say they care about me. I don't want to hear it. They want to take me to the doctor! I don't want to go to the doctor. No way I'm talking to some stranger!*

things to do

Family Doctor or General Practitioner

It's important to see your family doctor or a general practitioner for a check-up in case there is some physical or medical problem that is causing or worsening your depression. If there is such a problem, you may need to have it treated in order to feel better. It may be a problem that will get worse if it is not treated. In addition, your doctor can suggest other possible treatments like medication (see Chapter 8, *Medication*) or may refer you to a doctor who specializes in the treatment of depression, a mental health worker, or another kind of specialist.

Sometimes your family doctor may not feel like the right person to help you because:

- You don't feel that you need help or that anyone would want to help you.
- You are afraid of doctors.
- The family doctor treated you when you were young and hasn't seen you in a long time.
- He or she seems too busy to talk.
- You feel as if he or she won't listen to you, only to your parents, or will share personal information with others.
- You are afraid the doctor will want to get into other areas of your life that you don't want him or her to know about.

If these reasons or other reasons are keeping you from seeing your family doctor, you may want to talk with a counselor or an adult you trust about these issues, or you may want to take one of your supporters with you when you see the doctor. Perhaps you will want to find another doctor, one who didn't know you when you were younger.

If you don't have a family doctor or if you need to find a new one who you are more comfortable with, call the local hospital or mental health agency for a referral. You might also ask trusted people in your life who they would recommend. You may want to briefly visit new doctors to be sure you feel comfortable with them.

Before you go to the doctor, fill out "Information for the Physician." You may want to get a family member or friend to help you with it. It will give your doctor clues that will help her or him to figure out as quickly as possible why you are depressed and the best way to treat your depression.

information for the physician

How I feel (refer to Chapter 1, *Am I Depressed?* for ideas):

_____

_____

_____

_____

_____

I have recently had changes in (describe those that apply):

_____ Appetite or diet

_____

_____

_____ Weight

_____

_____

_____ Sleep

_____

_____

_____ Ability to concentrate

_____

_____

_____ Memory

_____

_____

_____ Bowel and urinary habits

_____

_____

I have recently had the following symptoms (describe those that apply):

_____ Headaches

_____

_____

_____

_____ Numbness or tingling anywhere (where?)

_____

_____ Loss of balance

_____

_____

_____ Double vision or vision problems

_____

_____

_____ Alternating times when I feel great and when I feel terrible

_____

_____

_____ Coordination changes

_____

_____

_____ Weakness in arms or legs

_____

_____

_____ Fever

_____

_____

_____ Nausea or diarrhea

_____

_____

_____ Fainting or dizziness

_____

_____

_____ Seizures

_____

_____

_____ Stressful life events, such as the loss of a loved one, rejection, school problems, family problems, or moving

_____

_____

_____

_____

_____

The kinds of foods I usually eat for breakfast, lunch, dinner, and snacks:

_____

_____

_____

_____

_____

My use of caffeine-containing substances (coffee, tea, chocolate, soft drinks):

_____

_____

_____

My use of alcohol or illegal drugs, either currently or in the past:

_____

_____

_____

My smoking habits:

_____

_____

_____

All medications and food supplements (like vitamins and minerals) I am using:

Medication and dosage	When used	Why
_____	_____	_____
_____	_____	_____
_____	_____	_____
_____	_____	_____
_____	_____	_____

Medical history (include all major illnesses and surgeries you have had):

_____

_____

_____

_____

_____

_____

Family medical history (include all major illnesses of your parents, brothers, and sisters, as well as other close relatives):

_____

_____

_____

_____

_____

_____

information

Health Care Specialists

Your doctor may refer you to a psychiatrist, who is a medical doctor, with additional training and experience in working with teenagers who are depressed. Your doctor may ask this doctor to work with her or him on planning your treatment or may ask this doctor to take over the care and treatment of your depression.

Depending on your history and how you feel, your doctor may refer you to other specialists, such as a neurologist, an allergist, or an endocrinologist. If your doctor makes such a referral, ask her or him what that doctor does and why you have been referred.

There are many other kinds of health care professionals whom your doctor may refer you to or that you and your family may decide would be helpful.

Mental Health Worker

Your doctor may refer you to a mental health worker, or you may decide to see one on your own. That person may be called a counselor, therapist, psychologist, or social worker depending on his or her education, training, and experience. These kinds of health care providers will help you work through problems in your life that may be causing or worsening your symptoms of depression.

The mental health worker must be a person you like and trust, one with whom you can share anything. If you don't like and trust the person to whom you are assigned, ask for a referral to a different mental health worker. Only you can choose the best person to be working with you.

The mental health worker may suggest family therapy, where other members of your family are included in your counseling sessions— sometimes just you and your parents, or sometimes including brothers, sisters, and other family members who live in your home. You can decide whether or not you are comfortable with this approach.

You may see a mental health worker once, several times, or many times, depending on what you and the worker feel best meets your needs.

What to Expect from Health Care Providers

You may want your health care provider to:

_____ Assess how you are feeling, and prescribe a treatment that you both feel would be helpful

_____ Be willing to try new approaches and ideas

_____ Be willing to use less invasive complementary ways of treatment like massage or acupuncture

_____ Be willing to talk with your other health care providers and your supporters

_____ Consider your own needs and preferences

_____ Listen well

_____ Be able to talk with you in a helpful and supportive way

_____ Be caring, accepting, positive, hopeful, encouraging, understanding, compassionate, friendly, supportive, and respectful

_____ Help you learn how to take good care of yourself

_____ Be firm with you, and keep you from hurting yourself when necessary

_____ Be easy to reach, and have someone available to help you if he or she is unavailable

_____ Have up-to-date information on how you can help yourself and on possible treatments

_____ Help you to care for yourself

_____ Be willing to admit mistakes, and do the best he or she can to make up for mistakes

questions to answer

Is there anything else that isn't listed on page 46 that I would like from my health care providers?

_____

_____

_____

Do my current health care providers meet these criteria?

_____

If not, you could discuss your dissatisfaction with them. If they are not willing to meet your needs, you may choose to work with someone else.

information

Choices about Health Care and Health Care Providers

It is up to you, working with family members and other trusted adults, to decide what treatment is right for you and which treatment strategies and supporters you are comfortable with.

Find mental health workers and other health care providers by contacting mental health agencies or organizations in your area or by asking trusted people in your life whom they would recommend. You could also find out about services in your area by calling the office of any physician or counselor. When you are depressed, it may be hard to do this. If it is, ask a family member or friend to do it for you.

things to do

- I will ask _____ to contact health care providers for me if I am not able to do it myself.

- You may want to interview possible health care providers before deciding which one is right for you. You have a right to do this and should not be charged for such interviews.

- The choice of health care providers is individual and personal. The health care provider who works well for one person may not be best for another.

- Sometimes girls feel more comfortable with a female doctor and guys feel more comfortable with a male doctor. Others find that this doesn't really matter. The choice is up to you.

questions to answer

I would prefer working with:

_____ A woman

_____ A man

_____ It doesn't matter to me whether I work with a man or a woman

It is sometimes hard to find good health care providers. You may live in an area where there aren't very many. You may have to work with someone even though he or she doesn't meet all of your needs. He or she may be the only person available in your area or who is approved by your health insurance plan. Do not work with anyone who treats you badly. That will only make things worse. Do your best to find someone else.

information

Bad Treatment from Health Care Providers

Although most health care providers have very high standards, as in any profession there are a few who treat their patients badly. Your health care provider should not:

- Judge, blame, or criticize you

- Make you feel inferior or lower your self-esteem

- Tell you what you must do unless you are behaving in a life endangering or self-destructive way, such as drinking or using illegal drugs

- Try to force you to probe into areas and issues you are not ready to address

- Encourage you to try harder or work on your wellness faster than you feel able

- Try to make you remember things you don't remember

- Betray your confidentiality by telling others personal information about you

When health care providers say any of the following to you, it doesn't help and, in fact, may make you feel worse:

- "Just call the center in the morning."
- "You are just feeling sorry for yourself."
- "Why are you so quiet?"
- "I know best."
- "Just get over it."
- "It's all in your head."
- "If you would just try harder, you could do it."
- "Are you trying to hide something from me?"

If any of these things happen to you or are said to you, or if you feel uncomfortable in any way, talk to your health care provider about the situation. If you are not satisfied with the response, look for another health care provider.

CAUTION:
A good counselor will never suggest or allow sexual or inappropriate contact or any contact that makes you feel uncomfortable. Get away as quickly as possible from any health care provider who suggests, encourages, attempts, forces, or claims any type of sexual contact to be necessary to working together. Leave immediately. Do not see this health care provider again under any circumstances. Tell your parents or another trusted adult what happened, and ask them to report the person to the state licensing board or whoever is responsible for such matters in your area. Also, stay away from a health care provider if he or she:

- Tells you to stop relationships with family members or friends
- Tells you to trust him or her completely
- Threatens you in any way or tells you not to discuss your session with anyone else

A strong team of skilled health care providers will be very helpful to you as you recover.

8 Medication

overview

The decision to use medicine to treat your depression is a *big* one. Don't try to make this decision alone. Your doctor, counselor, and parents can assist you in deciding whether or not you should use medications. Before taking any medication, you, your parents, and the prescribing physician should all agree that this is the right thing to do.

Don't ever take a medication because a friend offers it to you. It must be prescribed for you by your doctor.

Medication is never the only treatment for your depression. It should always be combined with a variety of other things that you and your supporters agree would be helpful, like counseling, diet, and exercise (see Chapter 7 and Chapters 9–17).

> *The doctor is talking to my parents about my taking medication. I wish she would talk directly to me. It's my life! Why do I need to take medication anyway? How is that going to help? If everyone just quit bothering me, I know I would feel better. They tell me I shouldn't take drugs. Now they want me to take medication! Isn't that the same thing as taking drugs?*

You may not want to take medications because you:

1. Are afraid of possible long- or short-term side effects

2. Are afraid the medications will make you feel weird and you will not be able to enjoy yourself

3. Are afraid the medications will affect such things as your memory, intelligence, coordination, vision, and digestion

4. Feel you are a failure if you have to use medications to manage your life

However, the medications may be essential to your well-being for either the short or long term.

? information

Deciding to Use Medication

Here are some important factors to consider when deciding whether or not to use medication to treat your depression:

1. If your depression is severe and you are spending a lot of time thinking about suicide or planning how you are going to kill yourself, medication may help to keep you alive until you feel better.

2. If you have some of the following symptoms and they are so severe that they are interfering with your life, are a danger to your health, are preventing you from going to school or work, and/or are stopping you from taking care of yourself, you may want to use medication:

    *   You have lost weight or your appetite.

    *   You can't sleep, or you sleep all of the time.

    *   You can't concentrate.

    *   You feel emotionally out of control.

    *   You stay away from other people.

    *   You feel like everything is hopeless.

    *   You have no energy.

    *   Nothing you think about doing seems like fun.

You and your supporters will have to decide if the risks and ill-effects of your depression are greater than the risks or side effects of the medication.

Antidepressants, like all medications, carry some risks. These include:

*   Unpleasant side effects like nausea, dry mouth, and constipation

*   Danger when used along with other medications

- Extreme danger if too much is taken at one time or if used with alcohol or illegal drugs

If there were an "ideal medication," you would not have to worry about whether or not to use medication. A perfect antidepressant would have the following characteristics:

- It would take effect quickly (so it wouldn't take too long to get rid of it if there were side effects but also so accidentally missing a dose wouldn't have a big effect).

- The doctor would be able to measure its level in your blood and know what level is most helpful to you.

- It would have no side effects.

- It would neither affect nor be affected by other medicines you are taking.

- It would not be dangerous if you took too much.

- It would help your symptoms of depression to go away.

No such medication exists at this time, but new medications that work better, more quickly, and with fewer side effects are being introduced all of the time.

Chapter 6, *Understanding Depression*, describes how the brain uses neurotransmitters to transmit messages in the brain. It is a complex balancing act. Most of the time, this complex balancing act works well. You are able to experience normal patterns of sleep and appetite, to feel alert and energetic, and to have normal sexual feelings. However, if your neurotransmitters are out of balance for some reason, you may experience depression.

Antidepressants work by affecting the release, reuptake, or breakdown of the neurotransmitters in the brain. The neurotransmitters they affect include norepinephrine, serotonin, and dopamine. The extent to which each antidepressant affects each of these nervous system messengers determines the side effects of the medication.

Kinds of Medication

Three kinds of medicine are used to treat depression. You should know which type you are using and why. (Often, if the first medicine you try does not help, your doctor may recommend trying another medicine from the same group before moving on to another group.)

Tricyclic antidepressants have been around the longest and are the least expensive of the antidepressants. They are not as popular as they used to be because they can cause irregular heart rhythms. Because of their effect on the heart, they can be very dangerous if too much is taken at one time or if they are combined with alcohol or other drugs.

Monoamine oxidase inhibitors have been found to be particularly helpful in treating the kind of depression where you sleep and eat much more than usual. They are rarely used for adolescents because of the strict dietary requirements associated with their use. New medications in this category are being developed that may not require such careful dietary control.

Selective serotonin reuptake inhibitors are the most commonly used antidepressants for adolescents. They are much more expensive than tricyclic medications but carry less risk of serious heart problems. They can also be helpful for other psychiatric problems such as obsessive-compulsive disorder, bulimia, or anxiety disorders.

things to remember

Taking Medications

Your doctor will instruct you on how to take the medication and help you make a plan for monitoring the effects of the medication. This may include regular office visits and certain testing procedures. Ask your doctor about this.

Different antidepressants take different lengths of time to help you feel better, from 2 days to 6 weeks or more. Most take 4–6 weeks for the full effect. You will not feel better right away.

Your doctor may suggest using several medications together to help you feel better and recover more quickly. Certain medicines when used together with antidepressants seem to increase the effectiveness of the antidepressant. When this is suggested, it is important to ask your doctor what he or she knows about this combination. Is it safe? How do the medicines affect one another?

Your doctor may suggest other medicines like antipsychotics, mood stabilizers, stimulants, or thyroid hormone replacement medications. As with the antidepressants, it is important to have your doctor explain to you why he or she is suggesting you use this medication; what the side effects might be; and how you, your parents, and your doctor can determine if the medication is helping.

Before taking any medication, you and your parents should have the information on the following page. Write it on the following page and keep it in a place where you can find it quickly. Also, ask the doctor for the information handout that comes with the medication.

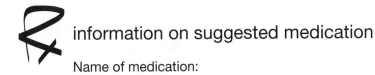

information on suggested medication

Name of medication:

_____

Why the doctor suggested this medication:

_____

_____

How long it takes to work: _____

What the medication does:

_____

_____

Possible side effects of this medication:

_____

_____

What medications to avoid if I am using this medication:

_____

_____

What foods to avoid, things to do, and things not to do when using this medication:

_____

_____

Other medications I am taking that I need to tell my doctor about (include all medications or herbal supplements you are taking for any reason):

_____

_____

_____

If you are taking medications for other physical conditions, ask your doctor how the medicines affect each other. Check with your doctor or pharmacist before taking any other medications. Some safe medicines when used in combination with other medicines can be quite dangerous. Even over-the-counter medicines like cough syrups or antihistamines can be dangerous when combined with certain antidepressants.

question to answer

How do I feel about using medications to treat my depression?

_____

_____

_____

_____

ASK YOUR DOCTOR OR PHARMACIST
ANY QUESTION YOU HAVE ABOUT USING
MEDICATION. DON'T WORRY ABOUT TAKING UP THEIR
TIME OR THAT YOUR QUESTION MIGHT BE CONSIDERED SILLY.

Your doctor and pharmacist are being paid to answer your questions. It is part of their jobs, and it helps to ensure that you will get the best possible results from using the medication.

Sometimes people may stay on antidepressants even after the depression is better to decrease the likelihood of becoming depressed again. That is a decision you have to make with your parents and your doctor.

next steps

If you, your doctor, and your parents agree that you should take medication, read Chapter 21, *Managing Medications.*

Again, it is crucial to remember that alcohol and illegal drugs (marijuana, hash, cocaine, acid, and so forth) will make you more depressed and interfere with the functioning of antidepressants.

THE COMBINATION OF ILLEGAL DRUGS AND
ANTIDEPRESSANTS, OR OF ILLEGAL DRUGS AND
DEPRESSION, IS VERY DANGEROUS AND CAN BE DEADLY.

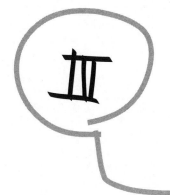

Things I Can Do to Help Myself Feel Better

9 Friends and Supporters

overview

When you are depressed, you need the friendship, advice, encouragement, and assistance of at least several other responsible people to help you get well and stay well. Although it is up to you to do the things that will help you feel better, you can't do it alone.

You may feel as if there is no one you can turn to when you are feeling bad. In fact, you may feel that there is never anyone you can ask for help; there is no one who cares about you. The adults in your life may seem to be too busy to be bothered, or they may be very judgmental and critical. You may have a hard time making and keeping friends.

In this chapter you will learn how to know who your friends and supporters really are and how to find friends and supporters if you feel that you don't have any or that you need more.

information

You need and deserve several friends or supporters who:

- You like, respect, and trust and who like, respect, and trust you
- You can talk to about your personal issues and know that they will not tell anyone else
- You can tell anything
- Listen to you
- Let you freely express your feelings and emotions without judging you or criticizing you
- Give you good advice when you want it

- Allow you the space to change, grow, make decisions, and even make mistakes
- Accept your good and bad moods
- Want to be your friend even when you are depressed
- Share information with you that they think would be useful
- Work with you to figure out what to do next in difficult situations
- Assist you in taking action that will help you feel better
- Encourage you
- May have interests similar to yours

questions to answer

What other things do I want from my friends or supporters?

_____

_____

_____

Do I have any friends or supporters who do these things for me? If so, I am very fortunate.

_____   _____

_____   _____

_____   _____

_____   _____

information

Friends and supporters *do not*:

- Give advice unless you ask for it
- Judge you
- Criticize you
- Put you down
- Tell you that the depression is your fault or that you should "get over it"

- Try to coerce you into doing things that don't feel right to you—like hurting someone else or driving too fast

- Tell you alcohol, illegal drugs, or sex would make you feel better

- Encourage you to take life-threatening risks

- Have you all figured out or have all the answers for you

questions to answer

Are there other things I don't want my supporters or friends to do?

_____

_____

_____

People who criticize you, judge you, or try to coerce you, among other things, are not really your friends or supporters. If you can think of anyone in your life who fits this category, list them here.

_____   _____

_____   _____

_____   _____

_____   _____

STAY AWAY FROM PEOPLE WHO TREAT YOU BADLY.
THEY ARE NOT DOING ANYTHING TO HELP YOU FEEL BETTER.
IN FACT, THEY WILL MAKE YOU FEEL WORSE.

It's best if some of your friends or supporters are responsible adults who can give you good advice when you ask for it and can take action for you when you need them to.

> *This depression—at least that's what they tell me it is—makes me feel cut off from everybody. I don't feel like talking to anyone. But last week I started talking to Alisha. She's always been a good friend. Afterward I felt a little better, not so alone. I think I might try talking to my Aunt Maria. She always seems glad to see me. Maybe she would understand and could give me some ideas on what to do. Maybe we could go to the movies.*

questions to answer

Which adults do I feel are my friends or supporters?

_____   _____

_____   _____

_____   _____

_____   _____

Other supporters will be friends who are your own age. They must be willing to listen and listen and listen. They are the people you will share good times and fun activities with. They are the people it is okay to be with without having to say anything. They must be people you have chosen to be your friends and supporters. Sometimes others will try to convince you who your friends and supporters "should" be. This is not okay. Your choice of friends and supporters is up to you.

Who are my friends and supporters?

_____   _____

_____   _____

_____   _____

_____   _____

If You Have Few or No Supporters

You may feel as if there is no one you can turn to, that you have no friends, that there is no one you can trust. According to one study, four out of five teenagers report feeling lonely sometimes or often because they have few or no friends. It's not hopeless. *You can take action to change the situation.*

Making friends is a skill like other skills—it can be learned. Having friends and spending time with other people can help keep you from becoming depressed.

You may have trouble making friends and developing supporters for a lot of different reasons. They may include the following:

• Others may read your discouraged mood as a lack of interest in them.

- You don't feel good about yourself, so you can't imagine that anyone would like you.
- You expect your friends to be perfect, so you can't find anyone who meets your standards.
- You are shy and don't know how to reach out to others.
- You are sensitive to any sign of rejection and react to it by giving up on the other person.
- You have not had the opportunity to learn how to make and keep friends and supporters.

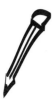

questions to answer

Which of these reasons may keep me from having the friends and supporters I need? (There may be several.)

_____

_____

_____

_____

_____

Are there any other reasons that keep me from having friends and supporters?

_____

_____

_____

things to do

The following suggestions will help you address the problems you have making and keeping friends. You may think of other ideas as well.

- If you don't feel good about yourself and it keeps you from having friends and supporters, refer to Chapter 16, *Raising Self-Esteem.*

- If you expect your friends to be perfect, and so you can't find anyone who meets your standards, refer to Chapter 17, *Changing Negative Thoughts to Positive Ones*.

- If you are shy and don't know how to reach out to others, practice being comfortable with others by joining a school club, church group, or community group.

- If you are sensitive to any sign of rejection and react to it by giving up on the other person, refer to Chapter 17, *Changing Negative Thoughts to Positive Ones*.

You may not have had a chance to learn how to be a good friend and supporter. It could be because your life has been very difficult. Maybe it is because you have a disability. Discuss this with a person you trust who you feel could be helpful. Tell this person that you have a hard time making and keeping friends and supporters, and ask him or her if there is something you are doing that is causing others to "turn off." Be prepared for the person to give you an honest answer because that is what you really need. They may say it is because:

- You don't look for friends in the right places.

- You are too loud and overwhelming.

- You never say anything.

- You are very shy.

- You feel bad about yourself.

- You don't listen when others talk to you.

- You have a negative attitude.

questions to answer

I think I have a hard time making and keeping friends because:

_____

_____

_____

_____

_____

_____

Once you have identified ways to help yourself make and keep friends, ask your supporters to give you suggestions, ideas, and support as you work on changing. Your supporters can also help you figure out how to address some of the other issues that you feel may be keeping you from making and keeping friends. The problem-solving activities in Chapter 11, *When Bad Things Happen*, will give you more ideas.

Help yourself make friends by:

- Joining an activity at school or in your community
- Getting involved in your church or synagogue youth group
- Practicing talking to people you don't know, like the clerk in the store or the other person waiting for the bus
- Listening closely to others when they are sharing with you— everyone likes a good listener
- Sharing with others openly and honestly
- Accepting yourself as you are
- Accepting others as they are without trying to change them

Try to avoid:

- Blaming others
- Becoming overly dependent on one or several other people

Good friends usually have some common interests and shared values. The things that are important to you should also be important to your friend. For instance, if you care about being honest and your friend is always shoplifting, you may need to let go of the friendship. If you are really interested in sports and your friend spends most of his time surfing the Internet, the friendship may not last.

A good friend or supporter doesn't have to be your age if he or she shares your interests and concerns. In fact, you may find that you enjoy spending time with an older adult or a younger sibling.

things to do

Where to Meet New Supporters and Friends

1. *Volunteer:* There are many agencies that could use your help like churches, schools, hospitals, youth agencies, environmental centers, soup kitchens, and the Red Cross. Ask your friends and supporters for ideas on places you could volunteer in your community.

2. *School groups and community activities:* What activities are available in your school and community? Would you like to get involved with activities like band, chorus, athletics, drama, and art or clubs like Boy or Girl Scouts, 4-H, and church youth groups? Is there something that interests you? Joining a group is a great way to meet new friends. Each school and community has its own special selection of groups, and most welcome new members. Check out your newspaper or ask your school guidance counselor for listings of activities and groups.

3. *The local teen center or recreation center:* Is there a local teen or recreation center? Do you feel welcome there? If not, why not? Is there something you could do about it?

It's hard to go to any of these activities the first time. You may feel out of place or like you are not really welcome. Everyone feels like that the first time. Go several times before deciding whether or not it is the right group, club, or activity for you.

Making the Connection

When you feel you have developed a special rapport with another person that feels like real friendship—that is, the person seems as interested and as eager to spend time with you as you are to spend time with him or her—make a plan to get together. The first time you meet could be a low-key activity like eating lunch together in the school cafeteria or walking to the bus stop. Also consider going for a bike ride, shooting hoops, or having a snack at a café.

As you feel more and more comfortable with the other person, you will find that you will talk more and share more personal information. *Make sure you have a mutual understanding that anything the two of you discuss that is personal stays between the two of you. Never make fun of what the other person thinks or feels.*

Don't overwhelm the person with telephone calls. Use your intuition and common sense to determine when to call and how often. Don't ever call late at night or early in the morning until you both have agreed to be available to each other in case of emergency.

Keep in Touch

Once you have met someone you like and who seems to like being with you, continue to make plans to spend time together. Each time you get together, end that time by making a plan for the next time you will be together. If something comes up you want to share in the meantime, you can arrange a get-together by telephone or in person, but always have something planned.

Key Points About Supportive Situations

- Let your supporter know what you want and need. For instance, you may say, "Today I need you to just listen to me."

- Spend as much time listening and paying attention to your friends and supporters as they spend paying attention and listening to you, unless you are feeling very depressed. Then, be sure you give them extra attention another time.

- Spend most of your time with supporters doing fun, interesting activities together. Don't be afraid to try something new.

- Take turns suggesting activities.

- Make a list of the things you like to do together to use when you are trying to think of something to do together.

- Keep regular contact with your friends, even when things are going well.

things to do

YOU MAY FIND IT HARD TO BELIEVE ANYONE WOULD LIKE YOU.

To increase your ability to understand that people *do* like you, try the following exercises:

- Ask a friend to tell you five things they like about you, then tell them five things you like about them. Do this often!

- Ask the other person to spend 5 minutes (use a timer) telling you why they like you. Then do the same for them. They can repeat the same thing over and over, like, "You are a warm, friendly, interesting person." Repeat this exercise often!

- Instead of saying to yourself, "No one likes me," say, "Many people like me." Before long, you will know that many people really do like you.

- Make a list of people who like you. Hang it in a prominent place in your room as a constant reminder. Add new names to the list as new people come into your life.

People who like me:

_____   _____

_____   _____

_____   _____

_____   _____

_____   _____

_____   _____

Keys to Keeping a Strong Support System

Once you have built a strong support system, how are you going to keep it strong?

1. Do everything you can to keep yourself well and stable. Make your wellness your highest priority. Others don't have a lot of patience with people who don't take good care of themselves and feel lousy a lot of the time.

2. Work on changing any bad habits you have identified that keep people from wanting to be your friends or supporters.

3. Be mutually supportive. Be there for others when they need you, as well as asking them to be there for you when you need them.

4. Have several friends so you don't wear out anyone when you are having a hard time.

5. Try peer or exchange counseling with your friends or supporters (see Chapter 14, *Peer Counseling*).

6. Make it a goal to find at least five good friends or supporters. Make a list of your support team members with telephone numbers. When you most need to reach out, it is hardest to remember who your friends and supporters are or to find their telephone numbers. Have copies of the list by your telephones, on your bedside table, and in your pocket.

support team members

Name	Telephone number
1. _____	_____
2. _____	_____
3. _____	_____
4. _____	_____
5. _____	_____

As you find new friends and supporters, update your list.

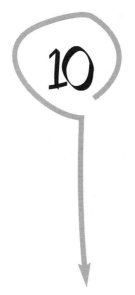

10 Avoiding Substance Abuse

overview

If you are using alcohol or illegal drugs, they will *worsen* your depression, even if they made you feel better when you first began to use them. They may also cause you physical harm, create havoc in your life, and put you at greater risk of killing yourself. In addition, the substances you are using may be addictive. This means that when you want to stop using them, it will be very hard. You may have to get special help to stop using the substance.

> *My Dad's been gone for a long time. He moved away, and we haven't heard from him for years. Every week, after he got his paycheck, he used to get drunk. Then, he would come home and make life hell for all of us. I always said to myself, "I don't want to turn out like that. I will never drink." My friends look like they are having such a good time when they are drinking. Maybe I should try it. Maybe it would help. It's really tempting, but I don't want to be like my father.*

information

Substance abuse can cause depression by:

- Affecting the chemistry of the body and the brain
- Causing you to do things you are later ashamed of
- Interfering with school and other activities

71

- Disrupting relationships with parents and friends (drugs and/or alcohol become the most important thing in life; they cause unusual and bizarre behavior that scares others away)

- Causing you to lose contact with others, like family and friends, who could help you find help or help you feel better. (You may spend most of your time with others who have similar problems or who can help you get the substances you crave.)

Substance abuse can cause a variety of health problems, such as memory loss and liver damage, and increases accidents of all kinds.

Depression can cause substance abuse. When you first use alcohol or drugs you feel better for a short while, so you use more alcohol or illegal drugs to help yourself feel even better. When you are depressed, you may be willing to try anything to feel better. The catch is that alcohol and drugs only make you feel better for a short time. Then, it becomes harder and harder to give them up.

Substance use can keep depression from getting better. How can it do that?

- If you are using antidepressant medications to treat your depression, the medications will not work as well, may not work at all, or could even become dangerous.

- It can make it harder for you to do the things you need to do to help yourself.

- It may have some of the same negative effects that depression does: decreased energy, decreased ability to concentrate, and decreased appetite.

- It may cause you to drop out of sports and other activities that could help you feel better.

- Self-esteem that may already be poor may get even worse.

- It can cause you to miss school, have a drop in grades, drop out of school, keep you from getting a job, cause you to lose a job, cause your boyfriend or girlfriend to break up with you, and so forth.

SUBSTANCE ABUSE INCREASES THE RISK OF SUICIDE.

Alcohol and drug use are always a problem. Substances don't make anything better; they only make things worse. It may feel like things are better initially, but that feeling never lasts. Substance abuse is *very serious* if:

- Your school work has deteriorated.

- You are having more fights with your parents.

- You find yourself using more than you intended.
- You have ever thought about hurting yourself.

What you can do to stop using or abusing drugs or alcohol:

- See your doctor or have a supporter help you get medical care.
- Contact a school counselor or an alcohol or drug counselor at your local community mental health center.
- Go to a meeting of Alcoholics Anonymous or Narcotics Anonymous (they will give you support and help you find the help you need).

If you have a good relationship with your parents, tell them about your problem. They would rather help you find solutions than have the problem worsen.

questions to answer

Substance abuse is a problem that may be causing or worsening my depression.

_____ Yes

_____ No

What I plan to do about it:

_____

_____

When I am going to do it:

_____

Who I am going to ask for help:

_____

_____

things to do

1. Stay away from:
   - People who abuse substances or sell illegal substances

- Places where people who abuse substances hang out
- Places where drugs and alcohol are easily available
- Events where there is heavy alcohol and drug use

2. Have a plan of things you can do if you feel tempted to drink alcohol or use drugs, for example playing basketball, calling a friend, drawing, writing in your journal, watching a good video or a favorite show on television, and reading a good book.

   Things I can do instead of drinking or using drugs:

   _____

   _____

   _____

   _____

   _____

3. Have a list of people you could call when you feel like having a drink or using drugs.

   People I could call when I feel like having a drink or using drugs:

   _____   _____

   _____   _____

   _____   _____

4. Work with an alcohol counselor on an ongoing basis.

5. Attend Alcoholics Anonymous or Narcotics Anonymous meetings on a regular basis.

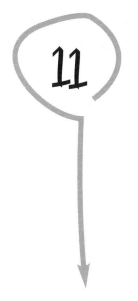

When Bad Things Happen

overview

Bad things happen to everyone. You cannot always keep bad things from happening to you. Sometimes the bad things that happen are your own fault and sometimes they're not, but you have to deal with them anyway. However, you can learn to deal with them in ways that keep you from feeling depressed.

> *My boyfriend broke up with me last week. He said I was always sad and he was sick of it. He said he wanted to go out with my friend, Tammy. Now I feel worse than ever. I bet they were talking about me behind my back. I'll never find another boyfriend, and I'll never trust my friends again. Life sucks!*

Generally, there are three kinds of bad things: temporary situations, ongoing situations, and life-altering situations.

temporary situations

Situations that are temporary affect you now but will not affect you for the rest of your life. They are the kind of things you "get over." Some days you feel worse about them than other days, but they gradually diminish in importance as you get involved in other activities. After a while they don't matter much at all. For example:

- You got a low grade on a test in a subject that you usually do well in, and you know your parents will be upset.
- Your boyfriend or girlfriend has broken up with you.
- You have damaged the family car.
- You have lost your part-time job.
- A friend made fun of or ridiculed you.
- A friend moved away.
- You had a minor brush with the law.
- You couldn't do something you really wanted to do because your parents wouldn't let you.
- You don't have enough money to buy the bicycle or car you really want.

questions to answer

Some bad things that have happened, or could happen to me, that have had or will have a short-term bad effect on my life:

_____

_____

_____

_____

You can help yourself to feel better and get over these bad things more quickly.

next steps

If you continue to feel bad about this situation after a week or two and find that you are thinking about it most of the time, you may want to talk to a counselor or supporter about it. The following chapters will help you:

- Chapter 2: *Getting Help*
- Chapter 7: *Getting Good Health Care*
- Chapter 9: *Friends and Supporters*

ongoing situations

Ongoing situations are serious circumstances that are affecting you now and have been affecting you for a while. These are things that you need to, or can, do something about or that will improve with time. For example:

- You are overweight or underweight.
- You are very late maturing physically.
- You have severe acne.
- You are very lonely.
- You have no money to continue your education.
- You are in a relationship with someone you don't want to be in a relationship with.
- You have an illness (i.e., mononucleosis, diabetes, herpes) or an injury.

questions to answer

Some bad things that are serious but that I can eventually get over:

_____

_____

_____

_____

To figure out how to improve these situations, try the problem-solving activity that follows. Use the example as a guide. Ask a friend, supporter, or health care provider to work with you on this activity if that feels right to you. It's easier and improves your chances of success if you work on one problem at a time.

things to do: problem-solving activity

One situation that is really bothering me:

_____

_____

Possible things I can do to improve or correct the situation:

_____

_____

_____

_____

_____

_____

Think about each one of these things carefully. Which ones are not possible? Put an *N* next to those. Which ones would be difficult to act on? Put a question mark (?) next to those. Which ones could you do right now? Put a *Y* next to those.

Now make a contract with yourself to do all the *Y* things. Pick a date.

By _____ (date), I will _____

_____

By _____ (date), I will _____

_____

When you have completed the *Y* things, go on to the more difficult (?) things. Make a contract with yourself to do those.

By _____ (date), I will _____

_____

By _____ (date), I will _____

_____

Now maybe some of the *N* things don't look so hard. If there are any you think you could manage, make a contract and take that action.

By _____ (date), I will _____

_____

By _____ (date), I will _____

_____

questions to answer

Now that I have completed these contracts, how has the situation changed?

_____

_____

_____

_____

_____

If the situation is still not as good as you would like, go through this process again. Following is an example of using this problem-solving method.

1. Write down one situation that is really bothering you.

    I really want to go to college, but I have no money and my parents can't afford to help me.

2. List of possible things you can do to improve or correct the situation.

    _____ Talk to my school counselor about the possibility of scholarships and student loans and/or financial aid.

    _____ Research possible scholarships in the library and on the Internet.

    _____ Apply for all possible scholarships.

    _____ Apply for student loans.

    _____ Take a year off between high school and college to earn enough money to go to college.

    _____ Work and go to college at the same time, taking fewer courses and taking longer to graduate.

    _____ Go to night school and work days.

    _____ Go to a community college for the first 2 years, where the courses are cheaper, and live at home.

    _____ Get a weekend or part-time job now.

3. Think about each one of these things carefully. Which ones are not possible? Put an *N* next to those.

    __N__ Go to a community college for the first 2 years, where the courses are cheaper, and live at home. (Parents don't have space for me, and community college does not offer courses in my field of interest.)

4. Which ones would be difficult to act on? Put a question mark next
    to those.

    __?__ Work and go to college at the same time, taking fewer courses
    and taking longer to graduate. (I would still have to pay full price
    for each semester at the school of my choice and living expenses
    would be the same, so I would end up spending more.)

    __?__ Take a year off between high school and college to earn enough
    money to go to college. (I am anxious to get started on college and
    living space would still be an issue, and it might cost more a year
    from now.)

    __?__ Go to night school and work days. (I think I would get too tired to
    do a good job, and some of the courses I want would not be avail-
    able at night.)

5. Which ones could you do right now? Put a Y next to those.

    __Y__ Talk to my school counselor about the possibility of scholarships
    and student loans and/or financial aid.

    __Y__ Research possible scholarships in the library and on the Internet.

    __Y__ Apply for all possible scholarships.

    __Y__ Apply for student loans.

    __Y__ Get a weekend or part-time job now.

6. Now make a contract with yourself to do all the Y things.

    By Nov. 1, I will talk to my guidance counselor about the possibility of
    scholarships and student loans and/or financial aid.

    By Nov. 15, I will research possible scholarships in the library and on the
    Internet.

    By Dec. 15, I will apply for all possible scholarships.

    By Jan. 1, I will apply for student loans.

    By Jan. 15, I will apply for a weekend job.

7. When you have completed the Y things go on to the more difficult
    ? things. Make a contract with yourself to do those.

    By Feb. 1, I will explore fully the option of working and going to college at
    the same time, taking fewer courses and taking longer to graduate.

    By Feb. 15, I will explore possible employment options and figure out ex-
    penses and living space options if I need to take a year off between high
    school and college to earn enough money to go to college.

    By March 1, I will fully explore the option of going to night school and
    working days.

8. Now maybe some of the *N* things don't look so hard. If there are any you think you could manage, make a contract and take that action.

By April 15, if other options haven't worked out, I will talk with my parents to see if we might figure out a way I could continue to live at home and go to community college. I would also see if courses I prefer would be available in the region.

9. Now that you have completed these contracts, how has the situation changed?

I am still waiting to hear about several scholarships. I have secured one. Student loans are available to cover some of my expenses, and I have a summer job lined up that should really help. If additional scholarship money doesn't come through, I have done the research and will proceed with one of the ? plans if necessary. I have worked things out with my parents so that if all else fails, I can live at home and go to a community college that is in a nearby town and has the courses I want.

next steps

You can get more help in how to deal with these situations by doing some of the activities in Chapter 4, *Helping Myself Feel Better Right Away*. That chapter will also tell you some things you *to avoid*.

You may also want to talk to a counselor or other supporter about it. The following chapters will help you:

- Chapter 2: *Getting Help*
- Chapter 7: *Getting Good Health Care*
- Chapter 9: *Friends and Supporters*

life-altering situations

Life-altering situations are things that are very serious and could affect you for the rest of your life. For example:

- A relative or friend has died.
- Your parents are getting divorced.
- You have a severe physical disability, like blindness or deafness.
- You have an illness that may end your life.
- Someone you are close to is dying.

- You are being, or have been, sexually, physically, or emotionally abused.

- You think you might be or know you are gay.

- You are responsible for someone else getting hurt or killed.

- You are addicted to alcohol or drugs.

- You are pregnant or you got someone else pregnant.

- You have been charged with a crime and must face the legal consequences.

questions to answer

Issues in my life that could affect me for the rest of my life:

_____

_____

_____

_____

things to do

These kinds of issues can make you depressed or make your depression worse. They are very serious. You need to take some action.

1. If possible, see a counselor (see Chapter 7, *Getting Good Health Care*).

2. Get support (see Chapter 9, *Friends and Supporters*).

3. Get further help by calling a telephone help line that specializes in assisting people with the kind of problem you have.

Although your situation is very difficult, you can learn to cope with it and enjoy your life. It's hard, but it's worth it. You are a very important and special person, and you deserve all the best that life has to offer.

How Do You Handle It if You and Your Boyfriend or Girlfriend Have Broken Up?

If your relationship with a boyfriend or girlfriend has just ended, you may feel overwhelmed with sadness or grief. You may have many of the symptoms listed in Chapter 1, *Am I Depressed?*. You may even feel as if you can't go on.

The following points will help you feel better and help you get through this difficult time:

- It may feel as if the terrible pain and loneliness will never go away. Remember, the pain from such a break-up will go away. You WILL feel better.

- Spend as much time as you can with friends and family members who you enjoy being with.

- Keep yourself busy doing things you love to do (see Chapter 15, *Creative Activities*). Soon you will be feeling much better.

questions to answer

Things I enjoy doing:

_____

_____

_____

_____

_____

things to do

KEEP YOUR LIFE WELL BALANCED
SO RELATIONSHIP ENDINGS WILL NOT DEVASTATE YOU.

Almost everyone goes through several relationships before they choose someone they want to spend the rest of their life with.

Be prepared for relationships to end. If you have a boyfriend or girlfriend, you may want to spend every possible minute with him or her. It is important that you still have other friends and other activities that you do on your own—activities that make you feel good about yourself. Don't give up your connections with your friends and your parents when you fall in love. Even though you would like to spend every minute being with or thinking about your boyfriend or girlfriend, make sure you spend time with other people.

? information

◆ Sex

Issues related to sex and sexuality may be very confusing for you. You are not alone. Sex is a very confusing topic for everyone in our society.

People in our society disagree and have confusing attitudes about such issues as:

- Sex before or outside of marriage

- Homosexuality

- Abortion

Often, adolescents who are confused by our society's confusion become depressed because they feel one way and are being told they should feel some other way. This may cause or worsen depression. It is important that you understand the following:

1. You shouldn't kill or hurt yourself because you think one way and someone else thinks another way.

2. If you are clear about how you feel, it is usually easy to find others who will support you. Check out numbers in your telephone book, the Internet, or ask your guidance counselor.

3. If you are not clear about how you feel, talk to a therapist, counselor, or other supporter who is willing to help you explore your feelings and decide where you stand.

To keep yourself from getting into difficult sexual situations that may worsen your depression, remember:

1. Safe sex is essential to prevent unwanted pregnancy and sexually transmitted diseases like AIDS and gonorrhea. If you are sexually active, make sure you or your partner is using a condom and that no blood, semen, or other body fluids are being exchanged. You can get more information on safe sex from your doctor, Planned Parenthood organizations, or AIDS groups. You may be able to find some information on the Internet.

2. Everyone has a right to privacy about sex and sexual matters.

3. Everyone has the right not to be abused; treated as an object by others; or be forced, seduced, or pressured in any way into any sexual activity.

Moving

Moving is difficult for everyone. It can be especially hard if you are a teenager and you have no say in the decision to move. When you move, you lose your friends, your school, your favorite places, and your sense of who you are and how you are supposed to behave. When you become depressed after a move, it's extra hard because, if you are not close to your parents, you don't have a support system to help you.

There are things you can do to help yourself get through this hard time:

1. If possible, keep up your connection with your old friends while you are making new friends in your new location.

2. Join activity groups in your new school such as sports, band, or theater. Your school guidance counselor can let you know the activities that are available and how you can get involved.

3. Volunteer to help out in your new community at the places where additional help is always welcome like the hospital, nursing homes, schools, and libraries.

4. Ask a teacher or guidance counselor to help you find a buddy—someone who will teach you about the new community and school.

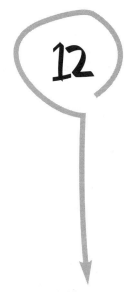

Diet, Light, Exercise, and Sleep

overview

Keeping yourself as healthy as you can is a good way to keep from getting depressed and, if you are depressed, to help you get better and to keep your depression from worsening. In this chapter, you will review some simple things you can do to take care of yourself. Remember, you are a very special person. You deserve to feel well.

> *I never have time for breakfast. I'm always tired, so I get up at the last minute and just about have time to get my clothes on before the bus comes. I grab something from the vending machines at school for lunch. By the time school is over I am starving, so I stop and pick up a hamburger, a large fries, and a shake. By the time my parents get home for dinner at 7:30 or 8:00, I want to be off with my friends. We have some chips, maybe some popcorn, and a few sodas. So that's what I eat! What does that have to do with the way I feel?*

 ## diet

To feel your best, try following these healthy diet guidelines every day:

1. Eat at least five servings daily of vegetables (about half a cup each). A big salad every day will help ensure that you are getting enough vegetables. Also include at least one or two servings of fruit.

2. Eat at least six servings of whole grain foods. Whole grain means that the food contains grains that are not ground into flour or bleached to

make the flour white. One slice of whole grain (dark) bread equals a serving, as does a bowl of whole grain cereal like granola, pasta, or brown rice.

3. Include some protein in your diet, like fish, poultry or other meats, eggs, cheese, or beans.

4. Include some dairy products in your daily diet, like milk, yogurt, and cheese. Limit or avoid the dairy products that contain lots of sugar, like ice cream and frozen yogurt. They are great for an occasional treat, but if you eat them often, you may feel worse. Don't get into the habit of getting an ice cream cone every day on the way home from school or work.

5. Replace artificial, refined, and processed foods like chips and canned spaghetti that are low in food value with foods that are natural and/ or raw.

6. Avoid or reduce your intake of:

   - Sugar (watch for hidden sugar in many prepared foods)

   - Foods that are high in saturated fats, like potato chips, french fries, and corn chips. There are some nonfat or low-fat snack foods available. Popcorn is a good low-fat snack.

   - Alcohol: it may make you feel better at first, but later you will feel much worse. It is also very addictive.

   - Caffeine (there is caffeine in coffee, tea, sodas, and chocolate). Caffeine makes you feel jittery and anxious and can interfere with sleep. This can worsen depression.

If you have trouble sticking with a healthy diet, some of the following ideas may help you.

- Ask your parents for their help. Ask them not to keep unhealthy foods in the house and to make sure you have plenty of healthy foods available.

- Carry a healthy lunch and snacks with you so you don't feel left out when others are eating.

- Avoid places that serve unhealthy foods like coffee shops, bake shops, and fast-food restaurants.

If you try to avoid eating, are very thin, eat and then vomit, eat too much and are overweight, or try as hard as you can to lose extra weight and can't seem to do it, ask your parents or your doctor for help. These can be very serious problems and need attention.

questions to answer

What problems do I have sticking with a healthy diet?

_____

_____

How could I solve these problems?

_____

_____

light

> *Holiday time again! Everybody is cheerful and busy. My parents don't understand why I am moping around. They keep telling me to have a good time. I've always hated the holidays. I never feel good at this time of year. I just want to eat and sleep. I wish everyone would leave me alone.*

Have you noticed that you are only depressed in the fall and winter or when there are several cloudy days in a row? You may have Seasonal Affective Disorder, more commonly known as SAD, if you experience several of the following symptoms during certain times of the year:

_____ Lack of energy

_____ Wanting to sleep a lot

_____ Difficulty getting out of bed in the morning

_____ Impatient with yourself and others

_____ Craving sweets and junk food

_____ Difficulty being creative

_____ Difficulty concentrating and focusing your attention

_____ Difficulty getting motivated to do anything

_____ Not getting as much done as usual

Scientists have found that exposure to sunlight helps some people who are depressed to feel better. Being outdoors in the light affects the activity of neurotransmitters in the brain.

CAUTION: Avoid looking directly at the sun or spending lots of time outside between 10 A.M. and 2 P.M. in the summer.

In the winter, the days are much shorter. You may get up and go to school or work in the dark and come home after dark. Sometimes you don't get out in the daylight at all.

More people who live in the northern climates (or in the southern hemisphere in the south) have SAD than those who live closer to the equator. If you live in the north, it is even more likely that SAD or lack of sunlight is causing part or all of your problem with depression.

things to do

There are some simple, safe things you can do to help yourself feel better if you think you have SAD.

1. Spend at least a half hour outside each day even on cloudy days. If you are at school or work, try to spend some time outside during your lunch break. Glasses, sunglasses, or contact lenses will block some of the sunlight you need. If you can't see well enough to go for a walk or be involved in some other outdoor activity without them, sit on a bench while eating your lunch or talking to a friend.

2. Gazing at the sky helps, but never look directly at the sun. The amount of light you get outside is enhanced by reflection off of snow and reduced by reflection off dark objects such as buildings and trees.

3. Keep your indoor space well lit. Have plenty of lights on. Let in as much outdoor light as possible. Spend as much time as you can near windows.

4. Check out Seasonal Affective Disorder on the Internet for more information and ideas on how to help yourself.

Some people notice almost immediate relief of symptoms when they begin increasing the amount of light they get through their eyes. It usually takes 4–5 days to work but may take up to 2 weeks. If you don't feel any better after 2 weeks of treatment with light therapy, your problem is probably not SAD. Tanning booths are not recommended for light therapy.

If these things don't help you enough, tell your doctor. He or she may be able to give you more information on how to treat this disorder.

If she or he doesn't know very much about it, ask him or her to refer you to a doctor who does. A physician who knows about light therapy will help:

- Diagnose whether you have SAD

- Make sure light therapy is appropriate and there are no other medical conditions that need treatment

- Work with you to develop treatment that fits your schedule and lifestyle

- Help you monitor how you are doing

- Provide additional ideas on how you can get more light

- Give you needed encouragement and support

 exercise

> *It's so hard to exercise these days. I just don't feel like it. I've always loved to go running. But now I can't even think about it. It's hard enough just walking to school. One thing I noticed though! Yesterday I felt better when I rode my bike to pick up a few things for Mom at the store. I'm going to try to take another short bike ride today.*

Exercise helps to reduce symptoms of depression. It is the cheapest and most available antidepressant. When you exercise, you will notice that:

- You feel better

- You sleep better

- Your memory and concentration improve

- Your symptoms of depression decrease

- You feel less irritable and anxious

- Your self-esteem will increase

It is difficult to exercise when you are feeling very depressed. Remember, even a few minutes of moving around will help. Do the best you can. If you can't do it at all right now, don't give yourself a hard time about it. Just begin to exercise as soon as you begin to feel a bit better. Listening to music while you exercise may help you feel more energized.

You can do the same kind of exercise every day or vary it according to the weather, what you feel like, and things you need to get done. You don't have to join an expensive health club (although it is a wonderful treat if you can afford it). It doesn't have to be strenuous. Even a walk helps.

What do you enjoy? Walking, swimming, skating, rollerblading, skateboarding, surfing, skiing, dancing—even outdoor chores such as cutting wood, raking, gardening, and playing with your pet can help.

questions to answer

What kinds of exercise do I enjoy?

_____

_____

_____

Make a contract with yourself.

I will exercise _____ (time of day), _____

(days a week), for _____ (length of time).

After you have fulfilled your contract for several weeks, give yourself a reward, like buying a CD you enjoy or going to a movie. Maybe your parents would help by giving you a reward. Tell them what you are trying to do, and ask them if they would be willing to help.

After I have exercised for at least 20 minutes every day for at least _____

days, I am going to:

_____ Reward myself with _____

_____ Ask my parents to reward me with _____

sleep

> *I wish I could sleep. I think I would feel better if I could. But in the evening I have the most energy—which isn't much—so I try to save that time to get my homework done. When I do go to bed, it seems like I don't sleep at all.*

A good night's sleep will help you feel better. Six to eight hours of sleep a night is enough sleep for most people. (If you sleep too much, you will feel worse.) Help yourself get a good night's sleep every night:

- Go to bed at the same time every night, and get up at the same time every morning. If you get to bed later than usual, get up at the same time anyway. You can take a nap later in the day.

- Avoid sleeping in. It will make you feel worse.

- Avoid or limit the amount of caffeine in your diet. Coffee and tea are not the only culprits. There is enough caffeine in chocolate, some soft drinks, and some painkillers to interfere with sleep.

- Avoid nicotine. It is a stimulant. If you cannot give up your smoking habit right now, avoid smoking 2–3 hours before bedtime.

- Avoid the use of alcohol. While it may help you fall asleep, it will disturb your sleep later and may cause you to awaken early.

- Eat on a regular schedule, and avoid a heavy meal prior to going to bed. Don't skip any meals.

- Eat plenty of dairy foods. They contain calcium that helps you sleep.

- Exercise daily, but avoid strenuous or invigorating activity before going to bed.

- When you are trying to get to sleep, play soothing music on a tape that shuts off automatically.

- Focus your attention on your breathing and repeat the words "in" and "out" silently as you breathe.

- Read a nonstimulating book or watch a calm television program before going to bed.

- Write in your journal about anything and everything until you feel too tired to write anymore.

- A turkey sandwich and a glass of milk before bedtime raises your serotonin level (one of those neurotransmitters in the brain) and makes you drowsy.

- A warm bath or shower before going to bed may help you sleep.

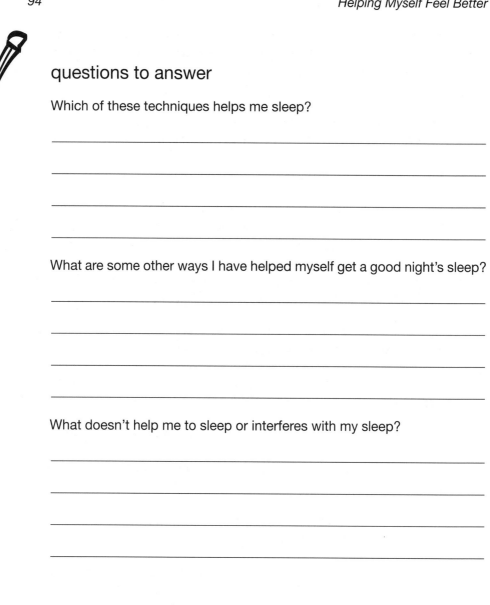

questions to answer

Which of these techniques helps me sleep?

_____

_____

_____

_____

What are some other ways I have helped myself get a good night's sleep?

_____

_____

_____

_____

What doesn't help me to sleep or interferes with my sleep?

_____

_____

_____

_____

13 Helping Myself Relax

I am tense and uptight all the time. Everyone notices it. My friends tell me to chill out. I'm not even sure what that means. I think I am just an uptight person. I never relax, never enjoy myself. My Dad is like me. It seems like he is always ready to explode, but usually he doesn't.

information

Many people use special relaxation and stress reduction techniques to help themselves feel much better. In order to use these techniques when you are depressed, it is essential to *learn how to relax when you are feeling well.* It is one of those things you learn and practice regularly that may even help keep you from getting depressed again.

Learning how to relax in our fast-paced society, where everyone expects us to be always working hard, is not easy. The best way to do it is to take a stress reduction and relaxation course. These are often offered free at hospitals or health care centers. Watch the newspaper for announcements.

You can also learn how to relax by practicing the exercises in this chapter.

things to do

In order to be effective, you must practice relaxation daily at a regular time. You will figure out for yourself the times when your house is most quiet and when you would be able to take a 15-minute break without interruption. Ask your family to respect this time by keeping quiet and not disturbing you.

Locate a space or several spaces in your home that are cozy, comfortable, and quiet where you can be away from the concerns of your life. It may be in your bedroom. Relaxing outdoors in a secluded place in the woods, in a meadow, by the ocean, or on a hilltop is also a good idea.

If you miss a time now and again, don't fret. Just do the best you can. Practice relaxing until it becomes second nature and until you can use it anytime you begin to feel nervous, tense, or irritable.

When you notice early warning signs that you are starting to get depressed, spend more time using your relaxation techniques, and do them more often during the day. At these times, it is helpful to use an audio- or videotape with a guided relaxation exercise.

Try some of the following relaxation exercises. See which ones help you feel better. (If any of these exercises make you feel worse, stop doing the exercise, and tell your doctor or counselor what you experienced.)

Breathing Awareness   Lie down on the floor with your legs flat or bent at the knees, your arms at your sides palms up, and your eyes closed. Breathe through your nose if you can. Focus on your breathing. Place your hand on the place that seems to rise and fall the most as you breathe. If this place is on your chest, you need to practice breathing more deeply so that your abdomen rises and falls most noticeably. When you are nervous or anxious you tend to breathe short, shallow breaths in the upper chest. Now, place both hands on your abdomen, and notice how your abdomen rises and falls with each breath. Notice if your chest is moving in harmony with your abdomen. Continue to do this for several minutes. Get up slowly. This is something you can do during a break at school or work. If you can't lie down, you can do it sitting in a chair.

Deep Breathing   This exercise can be practiced in a variety of positions. However, it is most effective if you can do it lying down with your knees bent and your spine straight. After lying down, scan your body for tension. Place one hand on your abdomen and one hand on your chest. Inhale slowly and deeply through your nose into your abdomen to push up your hand as much as feels comfortable. Your chest should only move a little in response to the movement in your abdomen. When you feel at ease with your breathing, inhale through your nose and exhale through your mouth, making a relaxing whooshing sound as you gently blow out. This will relax your mouth, tongue, and jaw. Continue taking long, slow, deep breaths which raise and lower your abdomen. As you become more and more relaxed, focus on the sound and feeling of your breathing. Continue this deep breathing for 5 or 10 minutes at a time, once or twice a day. At the end of each session, scan your body for tension. As you become used to this exercise, you can practice it wherever you happen to be in a standing, sitting, or lying position. Use it whenever you feel tense.

The Bracer   This is a good exercise when your energy is low. It will stimulate your breathing, circulation, and nervous system. Stand up straight with your hands at your sides. Inhale and hold a "complete natural breath" as described in the previous exercise. Raise your arms out in front of you, using just enough energy to keep them up and relaxed. Gradually bring your hands to your shoulders while contracting your hands into fists so that when they reach your shoulders they are clenched as tightly as you can make them. Keep your fists clenched as you push your arms out straight very slowly. Pull your hands back to your shoulders and straighten your arms out, fists tense, as fast as you can several times. Release your fists and let your arms drop to your side, exhaling forcefully through your mouth. Repeat this exercise several times until you feel its relaxing effects.

The Inner Exploration   Pick a part of your body on which to focus all your attention. Explore that part of your body in detail with your mind. What are the sensations in this part of your body? How does it move? What does it do? Is it tense? If it is tense, practice relaxing this part of your body. You may want to choose parts of your body that tend to be tense such as the neck, shoulders, jaw, forehead, or lower back. Or you may choose internal areas that tend to be tense such as the stomach or chest. Another idea is to focus on body parts that you rarely think about such as your toes, your elbows, or behind your knees.

Being Present in the Moment   Most of the stress in our lives comes from thinking about the past or worrying about the future. When all of your attention is focused in the present moment or on what you are doing right now, there is no room to feel anything else. When meditating, all of your attention is focused on the present moment. When other thoughts intrude, just turn your awareness back to the present. It is not necessary to be alone in a special place to focus all of your attention on the moment. Try doing it when you are feeling irritated waiting in a line, stopped at a street light, stuck in traffic, or feeling overwhelmed or worried. Notice how this makes you feel.

progressive relaxation

The purpose of this technique is to get you to focus on body sensations and how relaxation feels by systematically tensing and then relaxing muscle groups of your body. Make an audiotape recording of the instructions for this exercise so you can use it when you need to. Be sure you leave yourself time on the tape to tense and relax your muscles.

Find a quiet space where you will not be disturbed. You can do it either lying on your back or sitting in a chair, as long as you are comfortable. Close your eyes. Now clench your right fist as tightly as you can. Be aware of the tension as you do so. Keep it clenched for a moment. Now relax. Feel the looseness in your right hand, and compare it to the tension you felt previously. Tense your right fist again, then relax it, and again, notice the difference.

Now clench your left fist as tightly as you can. Be aware of the tension as you do so. Keep it clenched for a moment. Now relax. Feel the looseness in your left hand, and compare it to the tension you felt previously. Tense your left fist again, relax it, and again, notice the difference.

Bend your elbows, and tense your biceps as hard as you can. Notice the feeling of tightness. Relax and straighten out your arms. Let the relaxation flow through your arms, and compare it to the tightness you felt previously. Tense and relax your biceps again.

Wrinkle your forehead as tightly as you can. Now relax it and let it smooth out. Feel your forehead and scalp becoming relaxed. Now frown and notice the tension spreading through your forehead again. Relax and allow your forehead to become smooth.

Close your eyes now and squint them very tightly. Feel the tension. Now relax your eyes. Tense and relax your eyes again. Now let them remain gently closed.

Now clench your jaw, bite hard and feel the tension through your jaw. Now relax your jaw. Your lips will be slightly parted. Notice the difference. Clench and relax again.

Press your tongue against the roof of your mouth. Now relax. Do this again.

Press and purse your lips together. Now relax them. Repeat this.

Feel the relaxation throughout your forehead, scalp, eyes, jaw, tongue, and lips.

Hold your head back as far as it can comfortably go, and observe the tightness in the neck. Roll it to the right, and notice how the tension moves and changes. Roll your head to the left, and notice how the tension moves and changes. Now straighten your head and bring it forward, pressing your chin against your chest. Notice the tension in your throat and the back of your neck. Now relax and allow your shoulders to return to a comfortable position. Allow yourself to feel more and more relaxed. Now shrug your shoulders and hunch your head down between them. Relax your shoulders. Allow them to drop back and feel the relaxation moving through your neck, throat, and shoulders; feel the lovely, very deep relaxation.

Give your whole body a chance to relax. Feel how comfortable and heavy it is.

Now breathe in and fill your lungs completely. Hold your breath and notice the tension. Now let your breath out, and let your chest become loose. Continue relaxing, breathing gently in and out. Repeat this breathing several times, and notice the tension draining out of your body.

Tighten your stomach and hold the tightness. Feel the tension. Now relax your stomach. Now place your hand on your stomach. Breathe deeply into your stomach, pushing your hand up. Hold for a moment and then relax. Now arch your back without straining, keeping the rest of your body as relaxed as possible. Notice the tension in your lower back. Now relax deeper and deeper.

Tighten your buttocks and thighs. Flex your thighs by pressing your heels down as hard as you can. Now relax and notice the difference. Do this again. Now curl your toes down, making your calves tense. Notice the tension. Now relax. Bend your toes toward your face, creating tension in your shins. Relax and notice the difference.

Feel the heaviness throughout your lower body as the relaxation gets deeper and deeper. Relax your feet, ankles, calves, shins, knees, thighs, and buttocks. Now let the relaxation spread to your stomach, lower back, and chest. Let go more and more. Experience deeper and deeper relaxation in your shoulders, arms, and hands. Notice the feeling of looseness and relaxation in your neck, jaws, and facial muscles. Now just relax and be aware of how your whole body feels before you return to your other activities.

Guided Imagery

Guided imagery uses your imagination to direct your focus in a way that is relaxing and healing. Try the following guided imagery meditation.

Get in a very comfortable sitting or lying position. Make sure you are warm enough but not too warm and that you will not be interrupted by the telephone, doorbell, or needs of others.

Stare at a spot above your head on the ceiling. Take a deep breath in for a count of 8, hold it for a count of 4, let it out for a count of 8. Do that two more times.

Now close your eyes, but keep them in the same position they were in when you were staring at the spot on the ceiling.

Breathe in for a count of 8, hold for a count of 4, and breathe out for a count of 8.

Now focus on your toes. Let them completely relax. Now move the relaxation slowly up your legs, through your heels and calves to your knees. Now let the warm feeling of relaxation move up your thighs. Feel your whole lower body relaxing. Let the relaxation move very slowly through your buttocks, lower abdomen, and lower back. Now feel it moving, very slowly, up your spine and through your abdomen. Now feel the warm relaxation flowing into your chest and upper back.

Let this relaxation flow from your shoulders, down your arms, through your elbows and wrists, and out through your hands and fingers. Now let the relaxation go slowly through your throat and up your neck, letting it all soften and relax. Let it now move up into your face. Feel the relaxation fill your jaw, cheek muscles, and around your eyes. Let it move up into your forehead. Now let your whole scalp relax and feel warm and comfortable. Your body is now completely relaxed with the warm feeling of relaxation filling every muscle and cell of your body.

Now picture yourself walking in the sand on the beach on a sunny day. As you stroll along, you feel the warmth of the sun on your back. You lie down on the sand. The sand cradles you and feels warm and comfortable on your back. The sun warms your body. You hear the waves crashing against the shore in a steady rhythm. The sound of sea gulls calling overhead add to your feeling of blissful contentment.

As you lay here, you realize that you are perfectly and completely relaxed. You feel safe and at peace with the world. You know you have the power to relax yourself completely at any time you need to. You know that by completely relaxing, you are giving your body the opportunity to stabilize itself and that when you wake up you will feel calm, relaxed, and able to get on with your tasks for the day.

Now, slowly wiggle your fingers and toes. Gradually open your eyes and resume your activities.

next steps

The Relaxation and Stress Reduction Workbook (Davis, M., Eschelman, E.R., & McKay, M., 1999, Oakland, CA: New Harbinger Publications) and other self-help books will give you more information about stress reduction and relaxation.

There are many audiotapes that will guide you through relaxation exercises. These can be purchased at health food stores, book stores, and through many mail-order sources.

You can make these audiocassettes for yourself by taping yourself reading one of the relaxation exercises in this book with some pleasant music in the background. You can also tape yourself reading an exercise from some other resource book, or you can develop an exercise that feels right for you. You may find it easiest to relax using an audiotape when you are beginning to feel signs of depression.

14

Peer Counseling

overview

Peer counseling is a more structured way of getting the attention and support you need when you are depressed or when you are trying to cope with the stress of daily living. It provides an opportunity to express yourself any way you choose while being supported by a trusted friend.

Although peer counseling does not replace working with a counselor, therapist, or mental health worker, it is a wonderful technique that can help you express your feelings, understand your problems, discover some helpful action you can take, and even feel better. When used consistently, it is a free, safe, and effective self-help tool that encourages expression of feelings and emotions. It is very useful in addressing issues or problems identified in other parts of this book.

> *My friend and I tried "peer counseling." We were hanging around talking, and then she told me about it—how you divide the time (like an hour) in half and each of us talks, cries, whatever for half the time while the other person listens. Then, you switch. It was really neat. No one ever listened to me for that long before. And I love being able to say whatever I want without being criticized.*

information

Peer Counseling Sessions

In a peer counseling session, two people who like and trust each other agree to spend a previously agreed on amount of time together, dividing the time equally and addressing and paying attention to each other's issues. For instance, if two friends have decided they will spend an hour together, the first half hour is focused on one person, and the second half hour on the other person.

It is understood that the content of these sessions is between the two of you—no one else is told anything you talk about. Judging, criticizing, and giving advice are not allowed.

While most of us prefer sessions where we meet in person, they can be held over the telephone when necessary. Sessions should take place in a comfortable, quiet atmosphere where there will be no interruptions or distractions and where the session cannot be heard by others. Disconnect the telephone, turn off the radio and television, and do whatever is necessary to eliminate other distractions.

The content of the session is determined by the person who is receiving attention—the talker. The talker can use his or her time any way he or she chooses. The time may include eager talk, tears, crying, trembling, perspiration, indignant storming, laughter, reluctant talk, yawning, shaking, singing, wrestling, or punching a pillow. The talker may want to spend some time planning his or her life and goals. The only thing that is NOT OKAY is hurting the person who is listening or the talker hurting him- or herself.

Often, as the talker, you may find it most useful to focus on one issue and keep coming back to it despite feelings of wanting to avoid it. At other times, you may need to jump around from subject to subject. At the beginning of a session, a person may want to focus on one particular issue, but other issues may come up and take precedence during the session.

The person who is listening and paying attention needs to do only that—be an attentive, supportive listener. If the listener wishes, if it enhances the process, and if it is acceptable to the talker, the listener can ask questions (but the questions must be asked in order to help the person focus, not to satisfy the curiosity of the listener) or encourage expression of emotion. The talker, in turn, can ask the listener for specific things like:

- "Tell me what you like about me."

- "Pretend you are _____ (parent, friend, employer, and so forth), so I can safely practice telling her/him how I feel or what I want."

The listener must never demand anything of the other person. Full control must remain at all times with the talker.

In peer counseling, the expression of emotion is *never* seen as a symptom of a serious illness. Many of us feel that supporters view expression of emotion as meaning that something is wrong with us rather than as a vital part of our wellness process. You may have been treated badly for expressing emotion. Many of us have learned not to express emotion because it does not feel safe, thus interfering with our wellness process.

Contradiction

You may notice that during a peer counseling session you say the same negative things about yourself over and over again. This is not helpful and could even make your depression worse. When you realize you are doing this or the listener points it out to you, change the negative statements to positive ones (see Chapter 17, *Changing Negative Thoughts to Positive Ones*) and repeat these statements over and over again in the peer counseling session. Before long you will know that these positive statements are true and you will eventually feel better, even though at first it may make you feel worse.

Focusing Attention on the Present

1. When symptoms of depression are making you feel uncomfortable and keeping you from doing the things you need to do and the things you enjoy doing, you may want to focus your sessions on getting things back in order in your life and focus your attention away from issues in your past that you can't do anything about right now. Sometimes it helps to focus your peer counseling session on the present, putting your attention on pleasant things and your life as it is now.

2. At the beginning of a session the listener can reinforce the good that is happening in a person's life by asking him or her to share several good things that have happened in the last week (or day, or month, and so forth). This provides a starting point for the session.

3. At the end of the session the person who is listening brings the other person back to focus on the present by asking the person a benign question. The question can be a nonsense question or a question where you make up the answer.

   Sample questions:

   • What are computers for?

   • What color do you like the least?

   • What do you use couch cushions for?

- Where do you think the car that just went by is going?

- Why do people wear hats?

- Who is the most important person in the world?

At the end of a session (or when it is appropriate), it is useful to remind yourself to stay focused on the present by repeating the following affirmation:

I don't have time to focus on difficult issues. There are many things I would rather do (such as going for a walk, reading a good book, watching a video, petting the cat, going to a batting cage, painting a picture, and so forth), so I decide to focus my attention away from distress and onto pleasant and rewarding things in life.

questions to answer

Things I would rather do than focus on difficult issues:

_____

_____

_____

_____

_____

Many of us find it very difficult to focus our attention away from problems and issues when not doing peer counseling. Ongoing reminders will make this easier for you. Whenever you find yourself thinking about difficult issues, say to yourself:

I am going to stop thinking about my problems and _____

_____

You may have to remind yourself almost every moment to stay focused on the present when you are not peer counseling and when you are not using other techniques such as counseling, focusing, and writing in a journal to deal with your issues.

Don't be critical of yourself if this is hard for you. It is very hard for most people. It will improve with consistent practice.

Try peer counseling. It really helps!

15   Creative Activities

overview

Creative activities can help you feel better. Several are listed in this chapter. You can think of many others. Do those that you enjoy the most.

> *I love to write in my journal, but I am afraid someone will find it and tell my parents what I have written. Then, I would get in trouble, so I don't write about whatever I want. I wish I could. I think it would help. Maybe I could do it at Jen's house and leave it there.*

things to do

Journaling

People have kept diaries and written accounts of activities, events, and feelings for hundreds of years. Journaling, as we call it, is a good tool for dealing with various kinds of emotional upsets, including depression.

All you need to do is get some paper and a pencil or pen and start to write. Write anything you want, anything you feel. It doesn't have to make sense. It doesn't have to be real. It doesn't need to be interesting. It's all right to repeat yourself over and over. Whatever is written is for you only. It's yours.

You don't have to worry about punctuation, grammar, spelling, penmanship, neatness, or staying on the lines. You can scribble all over the page if that makes you feel better.

Don't fix your mistakes. Just keep writing. Draw or paste pictures or words in your journal if you want. Doodle. Anything goes.

Most people choose to keep their journal writings strictly confidential. No one should look at your journal if you don't want them to. You don't have to share your writings with anybody unless you want to. Put a note in the front of your journal that says, "This contains private information. Please do not read it without my permission. Thank you!" Have a safe, private place to store your journal, like in the bottom of your underwear drawer or on a high shelf. Other people in your household should respect your right to a private journal. Some people find it helpful and feel comfortable sharing writings with family members, friends, or health care providers. It's up to you.

You may want to set aside a time every day for journaling. It may be early in the morning or before going to sleep at night. Spend as little or as much time writing as you want. Some people like to set a timer. You can write in your journal anytime—daily, several times a day, weekly, before you go to bed, when you wake up, after supper, whenever you feel like it—the choice is yours.

You don't have to commit to keeping a journal for the rest of your life—just when you feel like it.

You can write at any speed you want, fast or slow. You can write as much or as little as you want.

You can write poems, paragraphs, verse, novels, novellas, fiction, reality, your autobiography, someone else's biography, wishes, fantasies, dreams, beliefs, loves, hates, and so forth. It can be similar each time or very different.

If you have had a hard time starting to journal, some of the following exercises may help you:

If my life could be any way I want, what would it be like?

_____

_____

_____

_____

_____

_____

What do I like about myself?

_____

_____

_____

_____

_____

_____

What made me feel good today?

_____

_____

_____

_____

_____

What made me feel sad today?

_____

_____

_____

_____

_____

What made me feel happy and excited today?

_____

_____

_____

_____

_____

_____

What is hard in my life?

_____

_____

_____

_____

_____

What makes me upset?

_____

_____

_____

_____

_____

What makes me happy?

_____

_____

_____

_____

_____

Who are my favorite people?

_____

_____

_____

_____

_____

_____

Here is a letter to someone I would like to tell off (but I know it wouldn't be wise) or to someone who is not available.

_____

_____

_____

_____

_____

_____

_____

Here is a letter to myself, pretending I am my own best friend.

_____

_____

_____

_____

_____

_____

_____

_____

The best thing that ever happened to me was:

_____

_____

_____

_____

_____

_____

_____

The worst thing that ever happened to me was:

_____

_____

_____

_____

_____

_____

Here is a list of all the reasons I want to be alive:

_____

_____

_____

_____

_____

_____

_____ I am committed to writing in my journal for _____

(how long), _____ (how often).

If you find that journaling is helpful, you may wish to get a copy of *The Healing Journey: Your Journal of Self-Discovery*, a workbook of journaling exercises by Phil Rich and Stuart Copans (John Wiley & Sons, 1998).

Music

> *Music is the greatest. I would listen to my music all the time if I could. I try to avoid music that makes me feel sad because I feel bad enough already. Sometimes just playing my drums really helps—especially if no one else is at home and I can really let loose.*

Both listening to music and making music may help you feel better. When you are feeling depressed, spend some time during the day listening to music. Have available tapes or CDs, or know the local stations that feature music you enjoy.

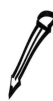

questions to answer

What kinds of music make me feel better?

_____

_____

Making music is also a good way to release feelings and pent-up emotions. What instrument or instruments do I like to play?

_____

Remember you don't have to play perfectly or even well to enjoy playing. You don't need anyone else to critique you. Just play for the sake of playing, for the fun of it.

Drums are great for this purpose. Put on some of your favorite music, and then just beat to the rhythm. Enjoy yourself. If you don't have a drum, find something that it is okay to beat a rhythm on, and use that.

_____ I am committed to using music to help myself feel better.

Art

> *I love to draw—well I did before I started feeling like this. I wanted to be an artist someday. But now I feel like I will never be able to do anything I want to do. I feel like nothing is going to work out for me. Maybe if I try drawing just a little bit each day it would help me feel better. I think I'll give it a try.*

information

Any kind of artistic expression you are comfortable with can help you to feel better. Maybe it's acrylics, water colors, oils, crayons, markers, colored pencils, charcoal, or stick-writing in the dirt. Perhaps you'd like to work with clay or one of the new synthetic clays. Maybe you'd like to carve something out of wood or even chisel away at a piece of stone— whatever feels good to you. Gather together the materials you need, and go to it. It helps to have the materials on hand, so when you feel like using them, they are available.

You are doing this to help yourself feel better and to let out feelings and emotions. It is not to benefit someone else. It is not a piece to be judged or graded.

questions to answer

What kind of artistic activities would help me feel better?

_____

_____

What materials would I need to get started?

_____

_____

Where and how could I get these materials?

_____

_____

_____ I am committed to using artistic activities to help myself feel better.

Other Crafts

The list of crafts that might help you to feel better is too extensive to list here. A few ideas include woodworking, knitting, sewing, building models, embroidery, cooking, photography, and metal work. You can think of many more.

questions to answer

What crafts might help me feel better?

_____

_____

What materials do I need to get started?

_____

_____

Where and how could I get these materials?

_____

_____

_____

_____ I am committed to using crafts to help myself feel better.

things to do

The hardest thing about these creative activities is getting started. Make a commitment to try an activity several times. If you enjoy it, make it part of your daily or weekly schedule. If you don't enjoy that one, try another. Keep working at it until you've discovered at least several creative activities you enjoy.

_____ I am going to try the following activities to see if I enjoy them. If I do, I will make them part of my daily or weekly activities.

Activity List

_____

_____

_____

_____

_____

_____

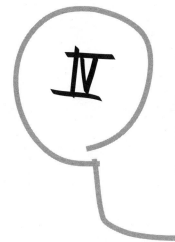

Things I Can Do to Maintain a Positive Outlook over the Long Term

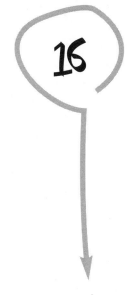

Raising Self-Esteem

overview

You deserve to feel good about yourself. Yet, many people report that they feel bad about themselves—have low self-esteem and lack self-confidence. Depression seems to make you feel even worse about yourself. Working on raising your self-esteem can help you feel better and may help prevent depression in the future.

> *I don't like myself. I never have. I feel like such a loser. I'm ugly. I act stupid. I'm not good at school. I don't think I was supposed to be born. I think my parents already had all the kids they wanted when I was born. Then, they got divorced. I am sure it was my fault.*

information

Raising self-esteem is often very difficult. It takes a long time and lots of persistence. Don't give up! It's well worth the hard work. Don't feel like you're alone. Other teens and adults will tell you that they have low self-esteem some or all of the time. Negative thoughts about yourself, especially when you have learned them from others, can be hard to let go of. Yet, if you do, you will feel so much better.

Low self-esteem and lack of self-confidence come from many sources. Many of us tend to blame our parents. In fact, many parents who were never taught good parenting skills may have contributed to this problem. However, sources of low self-esteem can come from many places—schools, television, the work place, social and religious institutions, friends, health care facilities, labeling practices, stigma, and prejudice. To feel better about yourself, you must have a strong sense of your own value as a person that is not dependent on others.

Physical, emotional, or sexual abuse, severe oppression, or being the victim of violent crime causes or worsens low self-esteem. If you have any of these issues, see Chapter 11, *When Bad Things Happen.*

questions to answer

How do I feel about myself right now?

_____

_____

How would I like to feel about myself?

_____

_____

Are there any people who you think contribute to your low self-esteem? If so, ask yourself, "Is this a person I should trust to determine my value?" Usually the answer is no.

NO ONE HAS THE RIGHT TO TELL YOU THINGS ABOUT YOURSELF THAT DAMAGE YOUR SELF-ESTEEM.

As a child, you were not able to understand that the bad things others told you about yourself were not true. You may have believed anything that was told to you by your friends or adults in your life.

things to do

Rename the Person Who Hurt You

It can be useful to give a name to whoever it was that gave you wrong information about yourself. This name can be anything, such as klutz, stupid, jerk, loser, bozo, good-for-nothing, worthless, and so forth. Close your eyes for a minute and find a name that most closely fits whoever was critical of you.

What would that name be? _____ It could be the actual name of a person who treated you badly. Does the name really fit? If it doesn't fit, keep working on it until you find a name that really fits. It is much easier to get rid of a source that has a name, rather than one that just exists in some general way.

Once you have found a name that works, use it to help you let go of negative thoughts or feelings about yourself. When they come up, say to yourself, "Oh, _____ made me feel that way." Then, let the thought or feeling go. You may have to repeat this many times to really get rid of those negative thoughts and feelings.

You may want to put the name on a piece of paper and put it in a balloon, then let the balloon float away. Or drop it in a brook and watch it float away. This helps you to feel like you are letting go of something.

Avoid People Who Hurt You

Include in your life only those people who treat you well and remind you from time to time that you are a good and worthwhile person. If the people in your life treat you badly, first try to correct the situation by explaining how bad their comments and actions make you feel about yourself. They may not have realized the damage they were causing.

I am going to tell _____ how the way he or she is treating me is making me feel about myself and ask him or her not to do it.

If the person keeps treating you badly, avoid that person as much as possible. This is sometimes hard if it is a family member, but do the best you can. If this is very hard for you, talk to your school guidance counselor, therapist, or doctor about it.

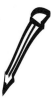

questions to answer

Is there anyone in my life right now who is treating me badly and telling me bad things about myself?

_____

How does it make me feel?

_____

_____

What am I going to do about it?

_____

_____

I am going to avoid contact with _____ because it is so damaging to my self-esteem.

The best way to keep yourself from being affected by negative comments, either from yourself or others, is to have a clear picture of who you are. Judge on your own whether there is any truth to whatever it is you are telling yourself, what another person is saying about you, or what a circumstance seems to be telling you about yourself.

things to do

Develop a positive statement of your worth. What are you really like? What kind of person are you? What wonderful things have you accomplished? Do it as if you were doing it for someone else. NO NEGATIVES ALLOWED. You will notice that there is a lot of space. Fill it up.

_____

_____

_____

_____

_____

_____

_____

_____

_____

_____

Make several copies of this statement. Keep them in convenient places, such as your bedside table, pocket, purse, bathroom mirror, refrigerator door, and journal.

Read the statement over and over to yourself. Memorize it. Then, whenever you start thinking negative thoughts about yourself, repeat this statement, silently if you are with others or aloud if you are alone. As you feel better about yourself, you may realize that you can change your statement of your own worth to make it even more positive. If you feel comfortable, ask a friend to read the statement to you several times. Spend time with people who help you to feel good about yourself.

things to do

I am going to spend time with the following people who affirm and validate me:

_____

_____

_____

People with depression have often developed negative perceptions of themselves. Focusing attention on negative and distorted thoughts about oneself contributes to depression. The thoughts worsen the depression, thereby causing more negative thoughts. These negative thoughts and the resulting low self-esteem can be addressed through cognitive therapy (see Chapter 17, *Changing Negative Thoughts to Positive Ones*).

next steps

_____ I am going to refer to Chapter 17, *Changing Negative Thoughts to Positive Ones*, and work on changing my negative thoughts about myself to positive thoughts.

Many people find that when they're repeating positive thoughts about themselves it brings up some emotion, usually sadness. Expressing the emotion by crying or telling someone about it helps to reinforce the positive thoughts.

Life circumstances can contribute to low self-esteem. They may include:

- Poor grades
- Physical disability
- Poor social skills
- Difficulty making friends
- Embarrassment caused by depression
- Family circumstances

When you are depressed you may think that some things are really bad that are not so bad. For instance, if you have a few pimples, you may feel as if you have a severe case of acne.

questions to answer

What circumstances in my life have made me feel bad about myself?

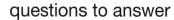

_____

_____

_____

_____

Should I let these circumstances determine my self-worth?

_____

Refer to Chapter 11, *When Bad Things Happen*, for ideas on how to deal with circumstances like these.

Do you feel guilty about something you have done? Does this keep you from feeling good about yourself? Perhaps you took advantage of someone, got someone pregnant or got pregnant yourself, broke the law, or damaged your parents' car.

things to do

The resulting guilt, especially if it is secret, can keep you from feeling good about yourself. Taking the following steps in your own behalf can help:

1. Tell someone or several of your supporters. Your counselor or doctor might be good choices.

2. Make amends in any way you can, like working to cover the costs of damages, paying for a stolen item, or apologizing to a person you have hurt.

3. Forgive yourself. Everyone uses bad judgment sometimes and does things they wish they hadn't. Try to let go of it. The guilt will diminish over time if you have done all you can to rectify the situation.

questions to answer

I feel guilty and ashamed because I:

_____

_____

_____

I am going to do the following things to try to make the situation better:

_____

_____

_____

I am going to forgive myself by:

_____

_____

_____

When I have done all I can to rectify the situation, I am going to forgive myself and try to let go of the shame and guilt.

things to do

Activities that Raise Self-Esteem

Try to do one or more of the following activities each day, especially on those days when you are feeling depressed or bad about yourself.

1. Write positive statements of your worth on a piece of paper. Carry the paper with you wherever you go. Repeat these statements over and over to yourself whenever you have time—while waiting at a street light or for an appointment, before going to bed at night, when getting up in the morning—as many times as you can.

    Positive statements of my worth:

    _____

    _____

    _____

    _____

2. Relax your whole body by progressively relaxing each part of your body, starting with your toes and working up. Then, repeat the positive thoughts in the first exercise over and over while you are in this relaxed state. Refer to Chapter 13, *Helping Myself Relax.*

3. Just as secrets you are ashamed of make you feel badly about yourself, secrets you are proud of can make you feel good about yourself. Begin to develop a "Secret Good Deed Account" that you don't tell anybody about—rake a neighbor's lawn, pick up trash in the park, send anonymous donations to a worthy cause you care about like the Humane Society, say nice things to your little brother. Be a better person than anyone imagines, and don't let anyone know.

    Good deeds I do or ideas for good deeds I could do:

    _____

    _____

    _____

    _____

    _____

4. Use your journal to write about changing negative thoughts to positive ones and activities you are doing to raise your self-esteem.

5. Make signs to post around your bedroom or living space that have positive statements about you that you have written. You could

make them fancy if you want, or you could make them with a computer. Read them several times whenever you see them.

6. Get together with a friend you trust and repeat positive thoughts about yourself over and over. Then, give them a chance to tell you positive things they are working on (see Chapter 14, *Peer Counseling*).

7. Get together with a supporter. Divide a block of time in half—for instance, with a 20-minute session, each person gets 10 minutes. Then, take turns telling the other person everything good about him or her. Just think, 10 minutes of compliments.

   I am going to try the compliment sharing exercise with

   _____

8. Regular meetings with a counselor you like and trust can help raise your self-esteem and self-confidence. Share with the counselor your list of positive affirmations from page 126.

9. Do something you enjoy that you know makes you feel better about yourself, such as painting a picture, taking a walk, playing a musical instrument, singing, reading a light novel, or going to a good movie.

   I enjoy:

   _____

   _____

   _____

10. Do something that makes you laugh, such as watching a sitcom on television, watching a funny video, reading a comedy, or getting together with a friend who has a good sense of humor.

    Some things that make me laugh:

    _____

    _____

    _____

11. Do something nice for yourself. Buy yourself something you have been wanting. Wear something that makes you feel good about yourself. Fix yourself a healthy lunch. Take a long hot shower.

Nice things I could do for myself:

_____

_____

_____

12. Do something special for someone else. Read a child a story, shop for a sick friend, send an "I'm Thinking About You" card to someone special, buy a friend an unexpected gift, volunteer at the local hospital, or mow a neighbor's lawn.

    Things I could do for someone else that would help me feel better about myself:

    _____

    _____

    _____

13. Pretend you are your own best friend. If you were your own best friend, what would you tell you about yourself, such as, "Take good care of yourself," "Eat right," "Do something fun," "Take care of your body," "You are a great person," and "I love you."

14. Make a list of your accomplishments—in a day, a week, a month, or your life. Give yourself credit for whatever you have done but not as compared with anyone else. Include things like completing kindergarten and learning to ride a bicycle.

    _____

    _____

    _____

    _____

    Post this list in a prominent place. Then read it every time you start thinking negative thoughts about yourself.

15. Set up a space to honor yourself, such as a bureau top or a wall in your bedroom. Then, fill the space with pictures of yourself, trophies, and other mementos. Spend a few minutes a day reviewing that space. Change the items as you feel like it.

_____ I am going to set up a place to honor myself

_____ (where).

I am going to include in this space:

_____

_____

_____

16. Put pictures of yourself in prominent view around your room. When you walk by each one, tell yourself something good about yourself.

   _____ I am going to hang a picture or pictures of myself in prominent places around my room.

   Pictures to include:

   _____

   _____

   _____

17. Ask for what you want and need for yourself. Advocate for yourself. Don't allow anyone to treat you badly. Don't allow yourself to be a victim! Be your own best friend! You deserve it!

   What I need:

   _____

   _____

   _____

   How I am going to get it:

   _____

   _____

   _____

18. Have a celebration. Celebrate that you got up, that you made the bed, that you went to school every day this week, that you wrote

a long overdue letter to a family member, that you made a difficult telephone call. Be creative. Then, give yourself a little party. Invite a special supporter, a family member, or a child to join you. Or celebrate by yourself. Have a good time. The celebration can be as long or as short as you want it to be.

Things I could celebrate:

_____

_____

_____

How I could celebrate:

_____

_____

_____

Activities like the ones described above, used consistently, will help raise your self-esteem.

DEVELOP A SENSE OF COMPASSION FOR YOURSELF.
LOVE YOURSELF AND TREAT YOURSELF LOVINGLY.
YOU ARE A WONDERFUL, UNIQUE PERSON.
BE GENTLE AND FORGIVING WITH YOURSELF.

next steps

Books to Read:

Copeland, M.E. (2001). *The depression workbook: A guide to living with depression and manic depression* (2nd ed.). Oakland, CA: New Harbinger.
Copeland, M.E. (1994). *Living without depression and manic depression: A guide to maintaining mood stability.* Oakland, CA: New Harbinger.
Fanning, P., & McKay, M. (1992). *Self-esteem.* Oakland, CA: New Harbinger.

Changing Negative Thoughts to Positive Ones

overview

People with depression often have a negative attitude and spend a lot of time thinking negative thoughts—thoughts that are not real, are not helpful, make them feel upset, and worsen their depression.

> *My mother says I am too negative. People say I am no fun to be with because I am so negative. My teachers say I have a negative attitude that is interfering with my school work. I can't help it. I don't like myself. I don't think anybody likes me, and I don't like my life. I have nothing to look forward to. And I feel really awful all the time.*

There are things you can do to get rid of these negative thought patterns. Start by discovering what your negative thoughts are. The negative thoughts or messages one gives oneself are often specific messages like ("I am a jerk," "You are such a klutz!") and short messages ("Stupid," "Idiot"). You usually believe them no matter how untrue they are. You repeat them to yourself in your mind very quickly, without thinking. They may include words like *should, ought,* or *must.*

Each person has her or his own negative thoughts. They are hard to turn off. You learned them somewhere, but you often can't remember where. They may include self-doubts such as, "I'm not smart enough to go to college," "I am not creative," "I am not likable," or "I am not good at anything."

Phobias are fears of specific objects or situations that seem unreasonably frightening like snakes, spiders, crowds, heights, airplanes, and darkness. Phobias are an example of another kind of negative thinking that gets in the way of wellness.

Figure out what your negative thoughts are. Carry a small notebook around for a day or two. Every time you become aware of a negative thought, jot it down in your notebook. You could also ask your friends or family members to help you identify your negative thoughts.

The following negative thought patterns may help you in identifying your negative thoughts:

Filtering   looking at one part of the situation without considering the whole situation. For example, if you missed one shot in basketball, you are a lousy player.

Polarized thinking   seeing things as either one way or the other with no in-between. For example, everyone in school loves you or everyone in school hates you.

Over-generalizing   reaching a general conclusion based on just one piece of information. For example, your girlfriend forgot to call you; therefore, she doesn't like you anymore.

Mind reading   making assumptions about how others feel without enough evidence. For example, the teacher called on someone else in class; therefore, the teacher thinks you are stupid.

Catastrophizing   expecting the worst will happen. For example, there is going to be a tornado, and you and everyone you like will be killed.

Personalizing   relating everything to yourself, including continually comparing yourself with others. For example, "I am not as pretty as my best friend."

Controlling   feeling either totally controlled by some outside force or feeling that you are personally responsible for everything. For example, feeling that your parents run your life or feeling like you are responsible for your parents' divorce.

Fallacy of fairness   thinking everything must be fair or equal. For example, if your sister can stay out until midnight, you should be able to as well.

Emotional reasoning   believing everything you feel must be true. For example, if you feel your boyfriend is interested in someone else, he must be interested in someone else.

Fallacy of change   assuming your happiness depends on the actions of others and that if they would change, things would improve. For example, "If my father would move back home, everything would be alright."

Blaming making someone else responsible for whatever is going badly. For example, dropping your radio and breaking it, then blaming the people who made the radio.

Shoulds operating from a rigid set of indisputable rules about how everyone should act. For example, "Everyone *should* like hard rock music."

Being right continually needing to prove that your view or action is right, even though evidence indicates that you are wrong. For example, needing to prove that a particular bicycle is best even though rating sheets and experience of others suggest it is not.

Perfectionism expecting never to make mistakes, to always be perfect. For example, expecting always to get A's on your schoolwork.

Some examples of negative thoughts that will worsen depression are:

- "I will never feel better."
- "I will never be able to play ball, skate, act, write (whatever it is you enjoyed doing) again."
- "I will never be able to go to college."
- "I am not smart enough for college."
- "No one will ever want to marry me."
- "I am ugly."
- "I am too fat."
- "I am stupid."
- "I don't deserve anything good."
- "Things will never get better."
- "I can't do anything right."
- "I am a complete failure."
- "I mess up everything."
- "I don't deserve to be alive."
- "I will never accomplish anything worthwhile."

These distorted thoughts 1) cause painful emotions such as worry, and depression and/or 2) cause you to have a hard time dealing with other people.

questions to answer

What are my negative thoughts?

_____

_____

_____

The next step in the process of getting rid of your negative thoughts is to *analyze your negative thoughts to see if they are true.* You may find it helpful to have a special notebook in which to do this work. Ask yourself the following questions. Really think about them. Be honest with yourself.

1. Are these negative statements true? Examine the evidence.

    Examples:

    - Since you got two A's, 2 B's and a C, how could you be stupid?

    - Your friend Mary calls you every night, and Linda calls you often. They must like you.

    - Your mother and your father have been fighting for years about issues that had nothing to do with you. You are really not responsible for their divorce.

2. Would one nice person say this to another nice person? If not, then should you be saying it to yourself?

3. Ask other people you trust. Say, "Am I really a jerk?" "Am I really a loser because I missed that basket?"

4. Examine the words you use, like *stupid* and *idiot.* Are they really appropriate? Remember, when you are doing this, you can only proceed with a positive attitude about yourself.

5. What do you get out of saying this to yourself? How does it help? How does it hurt?

Often, this step of analyzing a negative thought is all that is needed to get rid of it. However, with most negative thoughts, you will need to do more work to get them out of your consciousness for good.

The next step is developing positive statements that contradict the negative messages you have been giving yourself. Write down one or several of the negative thoughts you use most often, the ones that feel most important to get rid of. Write beside it a positive statement that is the opposite of the negative statement. Use the following rules to help you in this process:

1. Avoid using negative terms such as *worried, frightened, upset, tired, bored, not, never,* and *can't.* Don't make a statement like "I am not going to worry anymore." Instead, say something like "I will focus on the positive."

2. Use only positive words like *happy, peaceful, loving, enthusiastic,* and *warm.*

3. Substitute *it would be nice if* for *should.*

4. Always use the present tense, for example "I am healthy," "I am well," "I am happy," and "I have a good job" as if the condition already exists.

5. Use *I, me,* or your own name.

Examples of negative thoughts and positive responses:

Negative thought	**Positive response**
I will never feel good again.	I will feel good again.
I am not worth anything.	I am a valuable person.
It is not okay to make mistakes.	It is okay to make mistakes.
I want to die.	I choose life.
There is no reason for me to go on living.	There are many reasons why I should live.

Negative thoughts have often become so familiar that reinforcing positive thoughts takes persistence, consistency, and creativity. It takes several weeks to several months of reinforcement of the negative thought with a positive response to effectively change it. Commit yourself to spending some time each day, maybe just before dinner or before you go to bed, to work on reinforcing your positive statements. Reinforce positive responses by:

- Repeating them aloud or to yourself over and over

- Writing them down over and over again—10 or 20 times

- Asking someone you trust to read your positive responses to you

You can use other creative activities to enhance your work. Try making signs that say the positive response with markers or your computer and hanging them in obvious places around your bedroom. Read them to yourself every time you see them. You can think of other activities that will reinforce the positive statements.

Every time the negative thought comes up during the day, say "STOP!" to yourself and then repeat your positive response several times. Some people wear a rubber band on their wrist. Every time the negative thought comes up, they snap the rubber band and repeat the positive response several times. The rubber band method seems to work very well.

After you feel that you have gotten some of your negative thoughts under control, you can go through these same exercises with other negative thoughts. Or you may feel like taking a break from this work and coming back to it another time.

next steps

Refer to these books for more help in changing negative thoughts to positive ones:

Burns, D. (1980). *Feeling good.* New York: Morrow.

Burns, D. (1990). *The feeling good handbook.* New York: Plume.

Copeland, M.E. (2001). *The depression workbook: A guide to living with depression and manic depression* (2nd ed.). Oakland, CA: New Harbinger.

Fanning, P., & McKay, M. (1991). *Prisoners of belief.* Oakland, CA: New Harbinger.

McKay, M., Davis, M., & Fanning, P. (1998). *Thoughts and feelings* (2nd ed.). Oakland, CA: New Harbinger.

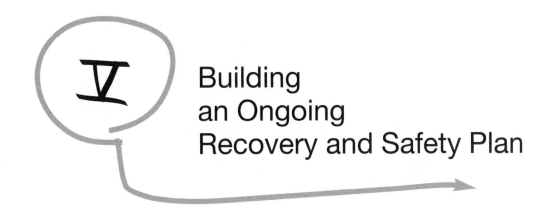

V
Building
an Ongoing
Recovery and Safety Plan

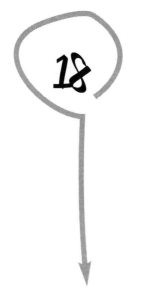

Wellness Tools

overview

In this book you have been introduced to many different ways that you can help yourself to feel better. In addition, you may have discovered some other safe things that you are already doing to help yourself feel better, and you may have thought about some other things you might do. It helps to make a list of all these things so that you can 1) refer to it for reminders of what to do when you are not feeling well and 2) develop a monitoring and action planning system like the one described in Chapter 19, *Monitoring My Moods and Preventing Depression.*

Although this may seem like a lot of trouble to you right now, it is well worth the time and effort. Many adults never take the time to do the things that make them feel better when they don't feel well or to do the things they enjoy. They even forget about them. They struggle along, not liking their life very much, until they get so ill or their life is so miserable that they have to do something to help themselves—or they don't bother and things just get worse and worse. You probably know adults like that, who are not very happy and who never take the time to do anything enjoyable.

But you are ahead of the game. You will be entering adulthood with a whole list of tools—a list you can add to whenever you discover a new tool—that you can use to 1) help yourself feel better when you feel depressed, 2) keep yourself from getting depressed again, and 3) make your life rich and rewarding. Your wellness tools are *your own choice.* No one else can tell you what you enjoy and what makes you feel better.

> *I know there are certain things I can do that always make me feel better—even when I am at my worse. Like last week. I felt like I just couldn't go on. Then my friend, José, came over. He listened while I complained. After a while, we were talking and laughing together, and we decided to go to a movie later in the week. By the time he left, I felt pretty good and even slept all night. Next time I am having a really hard time, I think I will call him or another one of my friends.*

developing your wellness toolbox

The following list of wellness tools includes ideas from many different people. If you think they would be helpful to you, put them on your own list. Then, add your own ideas. This list can be as short or as long as you want it to be.

Wellness Tools

- Spend time with a good friend or several good friends—list the names of your friends

_____

_____

- Spend time with a trusted adult—list the names of possible adults

_____

_____

- Call a friend or relative
- Call a help line or hotline
- Reach out for help from a health care provider
- See your doctor
- Go to see a counselor
- Talk to yourself in a positive way
- Go for a bicycle ride
- Swim

- Play baseball
- Skate
- Run
- Walk
- Go outside in the sunshine
- Watch television or a video—list those shows that make you feel better

_____

_____

- Listen to music
- Sing
- Play a musical instrument
- Play with a pet
- Read a story to younger sibling
- Eat something healthy that you like
- Get up at the same time every morning
- Go to bed a the same time every night
- Do something nice for someone else
- Help your parents with chores
- Call or send a note an elderly relative or friend
- Visit someone at a nursing home or in the hospital
- Go to the movies
- Read a comic or a book
- Play video games
- Draw
- Work with clay
- Sculpt
- Build something
- Make jewelry
- Sew
- Knit

- Write
- Cook
- Go to a support group
- Do some peer counseling
- Do a stress reduction or relaxation exercise
- Do guided imagery
- Journal—write in a notebook
- Get extra rest
- Take time off from your school and home responsibilities
- Take medications, vitamins, minerals, and herbal supplements
- Do something ordinary like washing your hair or shaving
- Surround yourself with people who are positive, affirming, and loving
- Wear something that makes you feel good about yourself
- Look through old pictures, scrapbooks, and photo albums
- Make a list of your accomplishments
- Spend 10 minutes writing down everything good you can think of about yourself
- Do something that makes you laugh
- Get some little things done
- Focus on and appreciate what is happening right now
- Take a warm bath

 things to avoid

You may also want to include on your list things that you want to avoid—that you know are not safe, are not helpful, or make you feel worse. Some ideas from others include:

- Being alone
- Drinking alcohol
- Taking street drugs or any medications that are not prescribed by *your own* doctor
- Having sex indiscriminately
- Doing anything careless or reckless
- Making major decisions when you don't feel well

- Going certain places in your area, such as places where others go to drink alcohol or where there may be drug dealers
- Getting overtired
- Watching the news or other shows on television with a lot of violence
- Spending time with people who treat you badly
- Eating junk food that has a lot of sugar, fat, salt, and/or additives (candy, cookies, cake, donuts, chips, fries, and soda)

My Wellness Toolbox

_____

_____

_____

_____

_____

_____

_____

_____

_____

_____

Keep your list of wellness tools in a convenient place—on your bureau, in your top desk drawer, pinned on your bulletin board, taped on a wall, in your wallet, and so forth—so you can refer to it when you need to remind yourself of things you can do to help yourself. You may want to make several copies to keep in different places so you always have one available. Add new tools to your list whenever you discover them. You can use your list to develop the monitoring and action plan described in the next chapter.

19 Monitoring My Moods and Preventing Depression

overview

If you have been depressed once, you may get depressed again. It is much easier to help yourself feel better when you are just beginning to get depressed than when you are deeply depressed. The monitoring system described in this chapter is designed to help you get better and stay better. The system will help others realize that you are starting to get depressed and may need help.

> My counselor offered to help me develop a system that would help me get better and stay better. It sounded like a lot of work, but I told my parents I would go see him every week, so I decided I might as well do it—then I wouldn't have to talk about myself so much. I thought I would never use this plan. But it's easy to do. I could have done it on my own. And it really helps. I notice I am having a lot more fun these days. My schoolwork doesn't seem so hard, and I don't feel tempted to drink to help myself feel better.

information

This monitoring system involves developing lists. Once you have developed your lists, check them every day—evening is a good time, but you can do it in the morning after you get up or any other convenient time during the day. It helps to do this daily review until you have been better for at least 4 months. Then continue doing it once a week. You need four things to get started:

1. Loose leaf binder

2. Set of five loose leaf binder divider tabs

3. Package of loose leaf paper

4. Pen or pencil (you could also develop these charts on your computer)

You can do this work on your own, but it always helps to have a friend or family member work with you as long as they do not tell you what you have to write.

things to do

Section 1: Daily Maintenance Activities

As you read this book, you discovered things you could do to help keep yourself feeling well or help you to feel better. Often, when people are having a rough time and need to do these things, they forget to do them or don't feel they can take the time to do them. Keeping track of what you do every day can help you get better and stay well.

On the first tab of a binder divider, write *Daily Maintenance Activities*, and put it in your loose leaf binder followed by several sheets of paper. On the first page, list those things you know you need to do for yourself every day to keep yourself well. It may include things like

- Eat three healthy meals a day, including breakfast

- Avoid junk food, sugar, caffeine, alcohol, and illegal substances

- Drink 6 glasses of water per day

- Exercise for at least a half hour

- Get at least a half hour of outdoor light

- Talk to a supporter

- Check in with my parents or some trusted adult for at least 10 minutes

- Spend at least 1 hour enjoying a fun, affirming activity

- Get at least 7 hours of sleep each night

- Take medications prescribed by my doctor

- Get up by 7:30 A.M.

- Go to bed by 10 P.M.

This list is just an example. Write one of your own that you think will work for you. *Review this page every day.*

On the second page, make a list of things you may need to do that day—things you don't need to do every day, but if you don't do them when you need to, they might cause you to get upset. The list might include things like:

- Call my counselor
- Call my doctor
- Spend time with my best friend
- Do peer counseling
- Clean my room
- Plan something fun for the weekend
- Talk with my parents

Section 2: Triggers

Write *Triggers* on the second tab, and put it in your loose leaf binder followed by several sheets of paper. On the first sheet of paper, make a list of things that, if they occurred, might cause you to become depressed or increase your feelings of depression. This list might include things like:

- Family friction and fights
- Fighting with or breaking up with your boyfriend or girlfriend
- Being teased, made fun of, or put down
- Feeling judged or criticized
- Being physically, emotionally, or sexually abused
- Situations that remind you of being treated badly
- A bad grade or grades
- A big disappointment like not getting accepted at the college of your choice or not getting a job you really wanted
- Rejection
- Feeling left out
- Being very overtired or having a physical illness
- Anniversaries of losses or certain holidays

On the next page, make a list of things you can do to keep yourself from feeling worse if one or more of these triggers happens. Some ideas include:

- Make sure I do everything on my Daily Maintenance Activities list
- Call a friend and ask them to listen while I talk about the situation

- Call my counselor

- Talk to my parents or other supporters about the situation

- Do some deep breathing

- Write in my journal

- Do some vigorous physical activity like playing basketball or bicycle riding

- Punch a punching bag

- Do peer counseling

- Listen to music

- Do a creative activity like drawing or painting

- Go for a walk in the woods

Review this list regularly, and when these triggers come up, do one or several of the things on your list.

Section 3: Early Warning Signs

On the third tab, write *Early Warning Signs,* and put the divider in your loose leaf binder followed by several sheets of paper. On the first page, make a list of early warning signs that you may be getting depressed. Everyone has different early warning signs of depression. Often, it is difficult to detect these early warning signs. It may be necessary to think back to the time just before you got depressed to discover what the early warning signs were. Ask family members and friends to help you discover changes in your behavior that may have indicated you were beginning to get depressed.

Following are some early warning signs of depression that others have experienced. They may help you discover your early warning signs of depression.

- Not enjoying activities you usually enjoy

- Not wanting to spend time with friends you usually like to be with

- Trouble getting to sleep or staying asleep

- Sleeping more than usual

- Not feeling like eating

- Wanting to eat more than usual, especially foods containing sugar or snack foods

- Feeling like you look fat or ugly

- Feeling more tired than usual

- Lacking energy

- Feeling more irritable and angry than usual

- Feeling like you are not worth anything

- Feeling like your situation is hopeless

- Crying a lot

- Having difficulty with schoolwork that is usually easy for you

- Having a negative attitude much of the time

- Having more trouble than usual getting along with family members

- Getting into trouble in school and/or at home

- Thinking about hurting yourself

You may find that you experience early warning signs of depression without stopping to think about what they mean. Thinking about them and reviewing them will help you become aware of your early warning signs so that you can take action right away to feel better.

If you notice that you have several early warning signs when you review your list, it is time for you to take some action to help yourself feel better.

On the next page, write down those things that you think will help you to feel if you are having early warning signs of depression. Some may be the same as those you listed under *Triggers*. You can list some things you *must* do like:

- Tell my parents

- Call my counselor

- Get some vigorous exercise

List some things that might be choices, like:

- Spend at least 1 hour doing an activity I enjoy

- Watch a favorite video

- Ask someone else to take care of my chores for a day

- Write in my journal for at least 15 minutes

- Take the dog for a long walk

Section 4: When Things Are Getting Much Worse

On the fourth tab, write *When Things Are Getting Much Worse*, and put it in your loose leaf binder followed by several sheets of paper. *When Things Are Getting Much Worse* means your symptoms have gotten worse but you are not yet to the point where you can't do anything to help yourself. You can still take positive action in your own behalf. Write down some symptoms that indicate your depression has gotten worse. They might include:

- Being unable to sleep
- Sleeping all the time
- Getting in lots of fights with family members and friends
- Wanting to be totally alone
- Not wanting to go anywhere
- Not doing the things I usually enjoy
- Thinking about ways I could hurt myself
- Not eating
- Crying all the time
- Grades getting much worse
- Unable to focus on school work or other work
- Substance abuse

On the next page, make a list of things you *must* do if some of these symptoms come up to keep the situation from becoming anymore serious. They might include:

- Ask my parents or other trusted adults to contact the doctor for me
- Ask my parents or other trusted adults to be sure I am safe at all times
- Arrange a special visit with my counselor right away
- Talk to at least two supporters, and tell them how I am doing
- Arrange, or ask a supporter to help me arrange, to take several days off from school or work
- Ask someone else to take care of my responsibilities
- Ask for extra time to complete difficult tasks or projects

The next section of this loose leaf binder will contain your safety plan, which will be described in Chapter 20, *Developing a Safety Plan.*

Become very familiar with the contents of this loose leaf binder. Check through it every day. Do the things on your Daily Maintenance Activities list. If any other symptoms come up, do the things you have listed that will help you stay well or will help you feel better.

Do everything on your Daily Maintenance Activities list every day.

Review the symptoms lists daily to see if you need to take action to help yourself get well and stay well.

After a while you may feel that some of the lists no longer meet your needs. Tear out those pages and make new lists that fit your needs more accurately.

Paste the list of supporters you developed in Chapter 9, *Friends and Supporters*, in the front or back of the binder for easy access.

next steps

You might want to read the following book.

Copeland, M.E. (2002). *Winning against relapse: A workbook of action plans for recurring health and emotional problems.* Dummerston, VT: Peach Press.

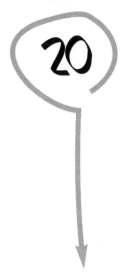

20

Developing a Safety Plan

overview

When you have been depressed and are finally feeling better, you may not want to think about the possibility of depression returning. However, depression sometimes does come back despite your best efforts to keep it away. It's a good idea to work with your parents and, if possible, your supporters and health care providers, to develop a safety plan. Then, the next time you are seriously depressed, they can easily do for you the things you need in order to get better as quickly as possible. Having a plan like this keeps you in control even when it seems as if you are out of control. This plan will help others know:

- When you need help

- Who you want to help you and who you do not want involved

- Medications you are using and why you are using them

- Kinds of treatments that are helpful to you and the kinds of treatments that are not helpful to you

- Specific instructions on what they can do to keep you safe, help you get through this hard time, and help you to feel better

> *I really don't think I will ever use this plan—especially now that I feel better. But I can see that it is a really good thing to have. Last time I was having a really bad time, my parents kept nagging at me and telling me I wouldn't graduate if I didn't do my schoolwork. After I finished the plan, I showed it to them. Now, they know that nagging makes me feel worse and makes it harder for me to do my schoolwork. It is better if they just ask*

me how they can help and listen to me without criticizing me or telling me what to do. They also know that a good meal, something like spaghetti with garlic bread and a salad, makes me feel a lot better.

things to do

On the last tab in the loose leaf binder you developed in Chapter 19, *Monitoring My Moods and Preventing Depression*, write *Safety Plan*.

1. Copy the form that follows on loose leaf paper.
2. Fill it in. You may want a supporter to help you with this form. This is a big task. Don't feel you have to do it all at once.
3. Make enough copies of your safety plan so that you can have one for your binder and one for each person you have listed that you want to take action for you when you can't take action for yourself. Give these people the copies. Review the plan with them so they will know exactly what you want them to do and when you want them to do it.

safety plan

What I am like when I am well:
(This helps you to remember what you are like when you are well and may be helpful to someone who doesn't know you and is trying to help you.)

_____

_____

_____

_____

_____

_____

_____

Symptoms

When I do the following things or have the following symptoms, I am so depressed that I can no longer be responsible for myself or do the things I have outlined in this plan:

(You might list things like using alcohol or illegal drugs, throwing furniture around, yelling a lot, crying all the time, threatening to hurt yourself or someone else, giving away your favorite things, not getting out of bed at all, not eating, and so forth.)

_____

_____

_____

_____

_____

_____

When I have any of the above symptoms, I want the following people to help me do the things I have written in this plan:

Name	Connection/role	Telephone number
_____	_____	_____
_____	_____	_____
_____	_____	_____
_____	_____	_____

I DO NOT want the following people to be involved in any way in my care or treatment:

Name	Why you do not want them involved (optional)
_____	_____
_____	_____
_____	_____
_____	_____

Medications

Doctor _____   Telephone number _____

Pharmacist _____   Telephone number _____

Allergies _____

_____

Medications/vitamins/health care preparations I am using and why I am using them:

_____

_____

_____

_____

_____

Please make sure I have and am taking or using these medications and health care preparations.

Medications I have used in the past that might be helpful:

_____

_____

_____

_____

_____

If you have any questions or concerns about my medications, please call my doctor right away.

What I want my supporters to do for me when I am experiencing these symptoms:
(Include things like make sure someone is always with me, do not leave me alone, let me express emotions, don't let me hurt myself, don't let me treat you badly, cook my favorite dish for me, get me my favorite

take-out food, give me things so I can draw or paint, feed the pets, call the school to get my assignments, arrange an appointment for me with my doctor or counselor, and so forth.)

_____

_____

_____

_____

_____

What I don't want from my supporters when I am experiencing these symptoms:
(Include things like don't yell at me, insist I exercise, make me eat if I don't want to, make me go to school, and so forth.)

_____

_____

_____

_____

_____

My supporters no longer need to follow this plan when I:
(Include things like get up and get dressed, go to school, call my friends, smile, and so forth.)

_____

_____

_____

I developed this document myself with the help and support of

_____

Signed _____ Date _____

Witness _____ Date _____

REVIEW YOUR SAFETY PLAN REGULARLY SO YOU ARE VERY FAMILIAR WITH ITS CONTENTS. AS YOU LEARN MORE ABOUT YOURSELF AND DEPRESSION, YOU MAY WANT TO CHANGE IT.

next steps

Refer to the following book for more information on safety plans.

Copeland, M.E. (2002). *Winning against relapse: A workbook of action plans for recurring health and emotional problems.* Dummerston, VT: Peach Press.

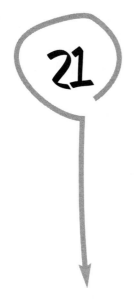

Managing Medications

overview

You, your doctor, and your parents can decide whether or not you will use medication to help reduce your symptoms of depression (see Chapter 8, *Medication*).

information

If you decide to use medication, there are some simple but important things you can do to ensure the safe use of the medication and to maximize the medication's effectiveness.

1. You still need to take very good care of yourself. You need to eat healthy foods, get plenty of exercise, get some exposure to sunlight, spend time with people who make you feel good about yourself, and take part in activities you enjoy.

2. Learn about the medication. Ask your doctor and pharmacist questions. Read the handout that comes with the medication. If you don't feel well enough to learn about the medication, ask a family member or supporter to do this for you.

3. Buy your medication from a pharmacist who has a good reputation and who knows you and from a pharmacy that has computerized record keeping systems. *Purchase all your medications at the same pharmacy* to avoid problems with medication interactions.

4. Never take any medication unless your doctor has prescribed and is monitoring it.

5. Ask the doctor who is prescribing your medication to contact all other doctors who are treating you before making any final decisions on medications.

6. Check with your pharmacist before taking any over-the-counter medication if you are taking an antidepressant.

7. Use the medication strictly according to the directions given to you by your physician or pharmacist, including having the regular blood tests required for that specific medication.

8. Many medications make you sleepy when you first start using them. It may not be safe to drive a motor vehicle or take part in athletic events. Check this out with your doctor.

9. Always consult your physician before changing the amount of medication you are taking or before you stop taking the medication. (Systems for changing medication and discontinuation are different for each medication and must be monitored carefully to avoid potentially serious reactions.) If you are having severe side effects and cannot reach your physician, contact another physician who your doctor has previously recommended as a backup for information on how best to deal with the situation.

10. Take the medication regularly. It is easy for anyone to forget to take their medication or to forget whether or not they have taken it. Special boxes are available that have a small compartment for each time you have to take your pill or pills (daily, hourly, and so forth). Using one of these boxes will help you to know that you are taking your medications regularly. A watch with an alarm or a small, inexpensive timer is a big help if you need to take your medication at a certain time each day.

11. Be completely honest with your doctor about whether or not you are taking the medication. If you forgot to take the medication several times, didn't renew the prescription on time, and so forth, tell your doctor to ensure that he or she can tell how the medication is working and so that any test results will be accurate.

12. Keep all medication out of the reach of younger brothers and sisters. They may be very intrigued by the plastic box, bottles, and pretty-colored pills. Store them well out of reach of children.

13. Most medication takes from several days to several weeks, depending on the medication, before you will feel any effect. Don't expect to feel better overnight. More likely, you will gradually notice you are feeling better. Because the changes are often gradual,

it is easy not to notice them. Keep a daily record of your symptoms so you can tell when you are getting better.

14. Medication side effects can often be reduced or eliminated by making some minor changes in the medication dosage, in diet, or in other habits. Ask your doctor for assistance.

> *My dad and I went to see the doctor. We agreed that if we found a medication that would help me feel better it might be a good idea for me to take it for a while. Maybe it would help me get my life back in order—catch up on my schoolwork and things like that. They stressed that medications are nothing to mess around with—that I would have to manage them carefully to be safe and to get the best effects. Dad said he would help me with it by reminding me to take it and checking in with me to see how I am feeling and if I am experiencing any side effects.*

things to do

Report the following medication side effects and any unusual feelings or symptoms to your doctor right away. They may be serious or dangerous. Don't wait!

- Blurred vision
- Rapid or irregular heartbeat
- Rash or itching
- Sore throat or fever
- Nausea and/or vomiting
- Slurred speech
- Stomach pains
- Insomnia
- Sleeping all the time
- Restlessness
- Confusion
- Lack of coordination
- Stumbling
- Jerking of arms and legs

- Ringing in the ears
- Impotence
- Changes in the menstrual cycle
- Large increase in urination
- Inability to urinate
- Nervousness, irritability, shakiness
- Fainting, seizures, or hallucinations
- Numbness of the hands or feet
- Swelling of the hands and/or feet

NEVER LET ANYONE ELSE TAKE YOUR MEDICATION.

NEVER USE ALCOHOL OR STREET DRUGS
WITH PRESCRIBED MEDICATION.

next steps

With good management, taking medication should be only a minor inconvenience in your life. If you have not done so already, read Chapter 8, *Medication*. If you have read that chapter, return to the chapter list in Chapter 5, *Using the Rest of this Book*, to decide how to proceed.

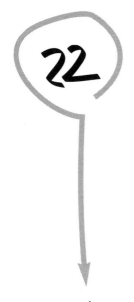

Avoiding Relapse

overview

If you have been very depressed, one of the riskiest times is when you feel worse again after making some improvement. You may become so discouraged that you give up hope and try to hurt yourself. Don't do it. Remember, depression is a treatable illness. **You will get better!** It won't be a steady process. As with most things, there will be times when you feel much better and times when you seem to be getting more depressed again. Try not to get discouraged. This happens to everyone.

> *I was doing so much better. I went back to work. I was thankful that Jay was willing to bring me back on because I really wasn't a very good worker before I quit. I brought my grades up. I was getting along better with my brother and my mom. Then, I started noticing that I was having trouble sleeping again. I didn't feel like going to soccer practice. I didn't feel like eating. But I don't feel so scared this time. I can talk to my mom about it, and she will understand and help me out. And I know lots of things I can do to help myself.*

information

This up and down is natural and part of the process of gradual recovery. At other times, you may be able to identify specific problems that are keeping you from getting better. Go through the following list and see if there is anything else you can do to help yourself. Review certain chapters of the book depending on what you learn from the list.

things to remember

Use the following list to keep you on track:

- There are many medical causes of depression. In order to seek out possible medical causes, you need a good physical examination and ongoing health check-ups.

  Have I been to a doctor recently? Do I like my doctor? Who could I ask to help me find a doctor and get better health care?

  _____

  Refer to Chapter 7, *Getting Good Health Care.*

- Sometimes medicines that help with depression can stop working. If you are taking medication, felt better at first, and now are feeling worse, contact your doctor to see if you need a higher dose of medication or a different medication.

  Do I need to check in with my doctor? I will call and make an appointment (when):

  _____

  Am I taking my medication according to my doctor's directions? What could I do to better follow my doctor's instructions?

  _____

  _____

- Are you being emotionally, physically, or sexually abused by anyone, including family members and peers? If so, your depression may recur or worsen. Talk to your guidance counselor or a trusted adult to resolve this situation.

  Is there anyone in my life who is not treating me the way I deserve to be treated? What could I do to stop this situation?

  _____

  _____

  Refer to Chapter 11, *When Bad Things Happen.*

- Difficult life events, which may include one or more of the following, may cause your depression to recur or worsen:

  1. Illness—your own or that of someone close to you

  2. Loss of a family member or close friend through death, separation, or rejection

  3. Moving

  4. Family upheaval and chaos

  5. Disappointment, like not getting into the college of your choice or losing your job

  What difficult situations am I dealing with? What am I doing or what could I do to help make these situations more bearable?

  _____

  _____

  _____

  Am I working out good solutions to problems as they come up? What could I do to solve my problems more appropriately?

  _____

  _____

  _____

  Refer to Chapter 9, *Friends and Supporters*, and Chapter 11, *When Bad Things Happen.*

- It is difficult to avoid substance use. Your friends may be using drugs and alcohol. They may try to persuade you to do the same thing. It is very difficult to resist. If you have previously had an alcohol or drug addiction problem, it is even harder. Try to remember how terrible depression feels, and that, although these substances may make you feel better for a little while, the long-term effects are dangerous and devastating. RESIST! If you are not able to resist, get help.

  Am I using alcohol or street drugs? What could I do to stop using these substances? Who could help me avoid drugs and alcohol?

  _____

  _____

  Refer to Chapter 10, *Avoiding Substance Abuse.*

- When you get busy or tired, you may neglect yourself. You may not eat right, stop exercising, and may even skip showers and other personal care tasks.

  Am I taking good care of myself, including eating healthy foods and getting plenty of exercise and light? What things could I do to take better care of myself?

  _____

  _____

  Refer to Chapter 12, *Diet, Light, Exercise, and Sleep.*

- Monitoring your moods is an important part of getting well and staying well.

  Do I have a system to monitor my moods to prevent depression? What system might work for me?

  _____

  _____

  Refer to Chapter 19, *Monitoring My Moods and Preventing Depression.*

- If the depression does get worse, having a safety plan in place will help minimize the effects of the depression and will help you get well more quickly.

  Do I have a safety plan? What is the first step I need to do in order to develop a safety plan?

  _____

  _____

  Refer to Chapter 20, *Developing a Safety Plan.*

- Being a teen with many body and life changes is stressful in itself. Add to that the increased expectations and responsibilities that you put on yourself and that others have for you. This stress can cause a recurrence of your symptoms.

  Do I have a lot of stress in my life? What relaxation exercises do I use to help myself feel better? What relaxation exercises would I like to try?

  _____

  _____

Do I use peer counseling regularly? Who could I ask to try peer counseling with me?

_____

_____

Refer to Chapter 13, *Helping Myself Relax,* and to Chapter 14, *Peer Counseling.*

• Time to do the things you enjoy is not just a luxury. It is a necessity. Be sure you have time each day for fun activities.

What are the creative, fun activities I use to help myself feel better and enrich my life? What fun things could I try?

_____

_____

Refer to Chapter 15, *Creative Activities.*

• Raising self-esteem is very important. One way to help raise self-esteem is to change negative thoughts to positive ones.

What am I doing to raise my self-esteem? What could I do? What are some negative thoughts that I have changed to positive thoughts? What are some negative thoughts that I need to work on?

_____

_____

_____

Refer to Chapter 16, *Raising Self-Esteem,* and to Chapter 17, *Changing Negative Thoughts to Positive Ones.*

If you can't find a cause or you need extra help and support to deal with a cause, let your parents, counselor, doctor, or other trusted adult know that you are having a hard time and need their help and support.

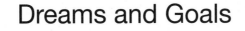

23 Dreams and Goals

overview

As a young person, you may feel like you have no control over your life—that the adults in your life are really in charge. You may have felt frustrated and even angry at times.

The adults in your life may not know whether to treat you as an adult or as a child. They may treat you as an adult sometimes and as a child at other times. This is very confusing for everyone. You, your parents, and other adults in your life will have to work together to get through this hard time as comfortably as possible.

However, this time in your life will be over very soon. You will be an adult and will be in charge of your life. Even now, you can make plans, think about your life dreams and goals, and even take some steps to help ensure that your life will be the way you want it to be.

You are setting yourself up now for your whole life—you are choosing a life path. *This path must be the path of your choice—not someone else's choice.* Others may try to direct your path. For instance, your mother may want you to be a doctor like your Uncle Fred. Or your grandmother may want you to be a teacher like your Aunt Jane. It may be important to your father that you go to college. In spite of all this input from other people—people whom you care about and who care about you—it is important that you do what you want to do, what feels right to you.

> *When I was young, I never thought about going to college. I didn't think I was smart enough, and my parents were too busy with illness in the family to even think about my future. And where would I get the money? I had planned to get some kind*

> *of job after high school—I wasn't sure what—to make enough*
> *money to support myself. Then, a school guidance counselor*
> *asked me where I was going to college. I was so surprised that*
> *she even suggested it that I did a double take. I said to myself,*
> *"Why are you shortchanging yourself? You can do whatever it*
> *is you want to do." I went to college. I was very successful*
> *there. I am doing the work I want and love to do, I have a nice*
> *home and family, and I am happy with my life. It could have*
> *been so different.*

Just because you have had depression as a teen does not mean you will
have depression all your life. It may or may not be an issue in the future. If it isn't, great! If it is, you know how to handle it. Don't let depression get in the way of how you want your life to be!

If you create a vision of what you want your life to be like, it may be
more likely to happen. The following questions may help you to think
about your future and decide if there is anything you need to do now.

DO WHAT YOU WANT TO DO. BE WHO YOU WANT TO BE.

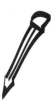

questions to answer

Career

What do I want to do for work or as a career?
(If you don't know right now what you would like to do for work, write
down your special abilities or talents and those things that you do now
that are most enjoyable to you. This may give you some clues about
what you would enjoy for a career. A career or guidance counselor could
talk with you about possible careers that make the best use of your abilities, talents, and the things you most enjoy doing.)

_____

_____

_____

_____

_____

_____

_____

_____

What do I want my life to be like?
(You may want to think about this question. Write as much as you want.)

_____

_____

_____

_____

_____

Education

Do I want or need to go to college? Where do I want to go?

_____

_____

Are there courses I need to take or things I need to do to get the education I want and need? If so, what are they?

_____

_____

_____

What do I need to do to make that happen?

_____

_____

Do I want or need to get some special training or experience? If so, what kind?

_____

_____

How and where could I get this training or experience?

_____

_____

Health

How important is good health to me and to meeting my goals and dreams?

_____

_____

What can I do to ensure that I will be healthy?

_____

_____

Leisure Activities

What kinds of things do I like to do for fun?

_____

_____

How can I make sure I will be able to do these things?

_____

_____

Family

Do I want to stay closely connected to my immediate family—mother, father, sisters, brothers, and so forth? How could I make sure I stay closely connected to them?

_____

_____

Although I may not have much control over this, do I hope to marry one day or be in a committed relationship? Describe that relationship:

_____

_____

Do I want to have children? How many children would I like to have? (Again, this can be unpredictable, but it is good to think about.)

_____

Home
What would my home be like?

_____

_____

_____

Where would my home be?

_____

Other Plans for Your Future
Other things that are important for me in my future:

_____

_____

_____

_____

_____

Roadblocks
What could keep me from doing the things I want to do in my life—things I may want to be careful about?
(Consider things like having an unplanned child, being addicted to alcohol or drugs, getting in trouble with the law, getting poor grades, and so forth.)

_____

_____

What I do to keep these things from happening:

_____

_____

As you go forward in your life, you may want to refer back to the important work you did in this chapter and in this book to keep you on track.

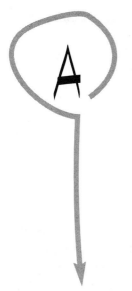# If a Friend Is Depressed

If a friend or someone you know is talking about suicide or you think they might be suicidal, tell a trusted adult right away. If the person you tell does not take action, keep asking until you find someone who will take preventive action. If you can't find an adult to help, contact your local mental health center or school guidance counselor. Don't stop searching for help until you have found someone who will take immediate action to protect your friend's life.

Don't let your friend be alone. If you don't feel safe being with him or her, get help from your parents, that person's parents, a guidance counselor, the police, mental health services, or some other trusted adult.

Friends may press you to keep their suicidal ideas a secret. YOU CAN'T DO THIS! Don't get into an argument about it or make any promises that you won't tell anyone. Your friend's life is at stake. Tell someone who can take action as quickly as possible.

spotting depression in a friend

Your friend may be depressed if he or she has one or several of the following symptoms:

_____ Looks and acts sad most of the time

_____ Is no longer interested in activities you used to enjoy together

_____ Has a different mood than usual

_____ Spends more time alone than before

_____ Seems very nervous or jittery most of the time

_____ Sleeps a lot

_____ Doesn't sleep

_____ Eats more than usual

_____ Has stopped eating

_____ Seems very discouraged

_____ Is very negative

_____ Doesn't make eye contact

(For additional symptoms, refer to Chapter 1, *Am I Depressed?*) If you check off several of the above items or you have noticed even one of the symptoms for a week or so, your friend may be depressed. Depression is very serious. As a friend, you have a responsibility to do something about it. You should be cautious in offering, giving, or getting help so that your friend does not get angry or deny that there is a problem. But depression is very serious. *You may have to get help for your friend whether or not he or she wants it.*

The first thing you *must* do is tell a trusted adult. It could be the friend's parent, a teacher, a guidance counselor, or a member of the clergy. Ask the adult what he or she is going to do, and make sure that happens.

There are also some very important things you can do. You will have to figure out which of the following ideas will work best in this situation:

- Tell your friend you have noticed that he or she is not feeling well, and ask what you can do to help.

- Spend extra time with your friend engaged in activities you enjoy together or simply listening without judging, criticizing, or giving advice (unless it's asked for).

- Share this workbook with your friend.

You will also need support for yourself when a friend is depressed or suicidal. Reach out to your parents, other trusted adults, and your friends. Ask them to listen to you and help you figure out what to do.

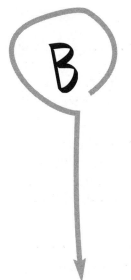

Information for Parents

Your teenager has given you these pages because he or she is depressed and needs your help to get through this difficult time. Adolescent depression is very dangerous. Your teen needs competent medical care right away. Ask your teen to share with you the symptoms of depression explained in Chapter 1, *Am I Depressed?*

Remember, your teenager's depression is not your fault, and it is not your child's fault. Depression is an illness like a cold or the measles. There are many different causes of depression, including certain diseases, hormonal imbalances, genetics, stress, medications, illegal drug or alcohol use, or poor diet. Your health care provider will help you and your teen figure out what is causing the depression and work with you to develop a plan for reducing and eliminating these distressing symptoms.

There are many positive things you can do to help your teen get through this very difficult time. But you can't do it alone. Reach out to others for assistance and support.

things you can do to help

- Help your child get the help he or she needs. This may include:

  1. Finding a doctor and a therapist

  2. Arranging for treatment

  3. Dealing with insurance issues

- Ask your teen what he or she would like you to do to help.
- Don't get angry with your child for being depressed.
- Listen—*without nagging or giving advice.* Just listen.

- Take your teen's pain seriously. Validate it. If your teen says he or she feels awful, tell him or her you are sorry he or she feels so bad and ask what you can do to help. Comments like "Snap out of it" or "It's not that bad" are NOT helpful and may make your teen more depressed.

- Remember, your teen is sick. Don't expect your child to be able to do the things he or she could do if he or she were well. You may have to take over some of your child's responsibilities, or ask others to help your teen until he or she feels well enough to do these things again.

- Learn about depression.

- In order to get the care and treatment your teenager needs, you may have to battle the following groups or organizations to get the support and care your child needs in a timely way:

  1. Insurance companies

  2. School systems

  3. Health care providers

  4. Treatment facilities

  5. Managed care providers

If your teen has recurring problems with depression, work with her or him and other people in her or his life to develop a plan of how you will respond to symptoms if they recur. Chapter 20, *Developing a Safety Plan*, guides your teen in developing a safety plan. Ask him or her to share this plan with you, and make a copy of it for your own reference.

If You Suspect Your Teen Is Suicidal

Many teens have thoughts of killing themselves. Many of them attempt suicide, and far too many are successful. If you suspect your teen is suicidal, you have to *take action immediately*. Take any suggestion of suicide seriously, even if the teen minimizes it. Ask your child if she or he is feeling suicidal. If your teen says he or she is, get help right away. Even if you think there's only a possibility your teen might be suicidal, get him or her help right away. You have to take action on his or her behalf, even if he or she does not want you to. It may be necessary to save your child's life.

Contact your local mental health agency or emergency services immediately for instructions and assistance.

Do not leave the teen alone. Your teen's assurance that he or she would never commit suicide is not sufficient. Teens often promise they will not try to commit suicide and then attempt it as soon as they are alone.

Remove, or have someone else remove, all dangerous weapons, fire arms, and medications from the home. Even after the danger has passed, it is wise to have such things stored outside the home, unavailable to your teen.

The suicide risk is increased if your teen has:

- Made previous suicide attempts

- Hinted about suicide in the past

- A history of depression

- A history of self-harming behavior or taking irresponsible risks

- Low self-esteem

- Used or is using alcohol or street drugs

- Suffered a severe loss

- A close relative who has committed suicide

Again, get help, and take action right away. There is no time to lose.

Things You Need to Do for Yourself

- Get help for yourself if you are having problems.

- Participate in family therapy.

- Attend a support group.

- Talk with supportive friends and family members.

- Take good care of yourself in every way.

As a parent, be aware that adolescents sometimes minimize their problems. What you observe may be even more important than what your adolescent tells you.

When Your Teenager Is Feeling Better

When your teen is feeling better, you can help ensure that he or she will not have a future episode by working with him or her in family therapy or supporting your teen in individual therapy. In addition, it helps to work with your teen to develop a plan to use in case the symptoms of depression return.

Recommended Reading

For more information on recovering from depression, you might want to read "Recovering your mental health: A self-help guide." This free booklet is available from http://www.mentalhealth.org or by calling 1-800-789-2647.

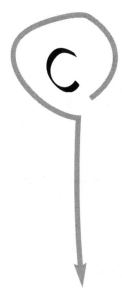

Important Telephone Numbers

An updated version of this appendix can be found at http://www.brookespublishing.com/recovering.

Al-Anon, 1-800-356-9996
Information and referrals to local chapters and meetings. Al-Anon is a support and discussion group for relatives of people with alcoholism. Spanish and French language services available.
e-mail: WSO@al-anon.org

Alcoholics Anonymous World Service, 1-212-870-3400
Information and referrals to local chapters and meetings.
Spanish language service available.

1-800-ALCOHOL
24-hour line for information and referrals about alcoholism.
Spanish language service available.
e-mail: info@adcare.com

Boystown National Hotline, 1-800-448-3000
24-hour hotline for children and parents for any problem.
Spanish language service available.
e-mail: Hotline@boystown.org

Center for Disease Control: National STD and AIDS hotline, 1-800-227-8922
8 A.M. to 11 P.M. Eastern Standard Time
Information on sexually transmitted diseases and referrals to local help.
Spanish language services available.
e-mail: hivmail@cdc.gov

Kid's Peace New England, 1-800-992-9KID

24-hour hotline for referrals to a residential facility in Maine that offers diagnostic and treatment services for youth younger than 18 with emotional and behavioral difficulties. Does not provide services for those who have mental retardation or have committed violent crimes or sex crimes.

National Alliance for the Mentally Ill (NAMI) Helpline, 1-800-950-6264

9 A.M. to 5 P.M. Eastern Standard Time
Information on medication and support group referrals for the mentally ill and their families.

National Clearinghouse for Alcohol and Drug Information, 1-800-729-6686

8 A.M. to 7 P.M. Eastern Standard Time
Ordering information for publications on drugs and alcohol. Books are free; audiotapes and videotapes are not. To reach a person, choose the "Information" option on the menu. Referrals also made to treatment centers.
Spanish language services available.

National Depressive and Manic Depressive Association, 1-800-826-3632

8:30 A.M. to 5 P.M. Eastern Standard Time
Educational information and resources, including local support group information.
Spanish language services available.

National Empowerment Center, 1-800-POWER-2-U

Information on psychiatric disorders and local referrals.
Spanish language services available.

National HIV/AIDS Hotline, 1-800-342-AIDS

24-hour line for information and local referrals.
Spanish language services available.

National Information Center for Children and Youth with Disabilities, 1-800-695-0285

9:30 A.M. to 6:30 P.M. Eastern Standard Time.
Information, legal advice, publications, and referrals for those working with youth with disabilities.
e-mail: nichcy@aed.org

National Referral Network or KIDSAFE, 1-800-543-7283 (1-800-KIDSAFE)

24-hour hotline with referrals for residential treatment centers and counseling.

National Runaway Switchboard, 1-800-621-4000

TDD: 1-800-621-0394, 24-hour hotline.

Help for runaways, suicidal youth, and their parents; messages sent to parents; gay and lesbian counseling; referrals for both youth and parents for counseling and shelters.

e-mail: Info@nrscrisisline.org

National Youth Advocacy Coalition, 1-202-319-7596

9 A.M. to 6 P.M. Eastern Standard Time.

Information and referrals for gay, lesbian, bisexual, and transgender youth. Will assist in setting up local support groups if none are available.

e-mail: nyac@nyacyouth.org

Planned Parenthood, 1-800-230-PLAN

Nationwide service for referrals to clinics. 24-hour line for recorded information on sexuality and reproductive health issues. To reach a person for a referral to a local clinic, call during the day (business hours vary).

Recovery Options, 1-800-NOABUSE

7 A.M. to 7 P.M. Pacific Standard Time.

Only crisis calls taken after hours. Information and referrals for anyone with a substance abuse or a psychiatric problem.

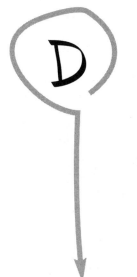

Information for a Friend

I am giving this to you to help you learn about my depression, so you can help me if I need you to. As you probably know already, depression is when people are so sad that it affects how their body and brain work. Depression is caused by a combination of difficult things in people's lives and by certain chemical imbalances in their body. The sad things in people's lives affect their brain chemistry, and when their brain chemistry changes, it interferes with the way their body and brain usually function. They may have trouble getting to sleep, may no longer be able to enjoy things that used to be fun, may feel uncomfortable around other people, may not feel like eating, may have trouble concentrating, may be irritable or cry a lot, may feel bad about themselves, and may even think about hurting themselves or killing themselves.

People with depression do get better. Both medication and therapy have been shown to help people get better. Other things that help people get better are exercise, spending time with friends, and doing things that help them feel better about themselves.

Some things make it hard for people to get better from depression. Using alcohol and drugs can cause or maintain the chemical imbalances that lead to depression. Alcohol and drugs also keep antidepressant medications from working and can be dangerous if combined with some antidepressant medications.

Even when people with depression are getting better, there can be ups and downs, particularly if sad or upsetting things happen while they are recovering. When people have thought about hurting themselves in the past, it is important for them to develop a safety plan to make sure they do not hurt themselves or try to kill themselves if they become upset. When they develop their safety plan, it is important for them to have people they know and trust that they can contact if they feel like hurting themselves.

If a friend tells you he or she is thinking of hurting him- or herself, it is important that you know what to do to help your friend. First, don't try to do it all yourself. If a friend is thinking about hurting him- or herself, you need to share that information with an adult who can help you help your friend. Depending on who you can reach, you may want to talk with your friend's parents, counselor or therapist, doctor, or psychiatrist, or a hospital emergency room, the police, a 911 operator, or an emergency 800 number such as the Boystown National hotline at 1 (800) 448-3000.

Besides helping keep your friends safe, other things you can do when friends are depressed are to spend some extra time with them, to get involved in activities that you enjoy doing together, to listen to them without judging or criticizing or giving advice (unless it is asked for), or to get some exercise with them such as going for walks or hikes together.

Help us make this book better!

We would love your suggestions for making this book more helpful to other teenagers who are struggling with depression. Please cut out this form. Fill it out, and mail it by folding it over, taping it shut, and putting a stamp on the back. An on-line version of this form can be found at http://www.brookespublishing.com/recovering. You may also photocopy this form and send it in an envelope to

Brookes Publishing Co.
Post Office Box 10624
Baltimore, MD 21285

1. Was this book helpful to you?   Yes   No

2. What was most helpful? _____
   _____
   _____

3. Are there other things we should include in the book? _____
   _____
   _____

4. Are there things we could change to make the book more helpful? _____
   _____
   _____

5. What things were most helpful in dealing with your depression? _____
   _____
   _____

6. How did you get a copy of this book?

   ___ Bought it at a bookstore   ___ Parents bought it for me
   ___ Borrowed it from a friend   ___ Therapist suggested it
   ___ Found it in my school library   ___ School guidance counselor gave it to me
   ___ Ordered it from a book catalog
        Which catalog? _____
   ___ Found it on the Internet
        Which web site? _____

7. Can you think of ways we can help get this book to other teenagers who could benefit from it? _____
   _____
   _____

Thank you for your help. We wish you well in your depression self-management and hope you assemble a great team to help you.

Mary Ellen Copeland
Stu Copans

Brookes Publishing Co.

Post Office Box 10624

Baltimore, MD 21285

RE: Recovering from Depression